Kriya Yoga and Turiya

A Comprehensive Guide to Kundalini Awakening, Yoga Asanas, Mudras, Meditation, Pranayama, Hindu Philosophy, Shiva, and Shakti

© **Copyright 2024 - All rights reserved.**

The content contained within this book may not be reproduced, duplicated, or transmitted without direct written permission from the author or the publisher.

Under no circumstances will any blame or legal responsibility be held against the publisher, or author, for any damages, reparation, or monetary loss due to the information contained within this book, either directly or indirectly.

Legal Notice:

This book is copyright protected. It is only for personal use. You cannot amend, distribute, sell, use, quote, or paraphrase any part, or the content within this book, without the consent of the author or publisher.

Disclaimer Notice:

Please note the information contained within this document is for educational and entertainment purposes only. All effort has been executed to present accurate, up-to-date, reliable, and complete information. No warranties of any kind are declared or implied. Readers acknowledge that the author is not engaging in the rendering of legal, financial, medical, or professional advice. The content within this book has been derived from various sources. Please consult a licensed professional before attempting any techniques outlined in this book.

By reading this document, the reader agrees that under no circumstances is the author responsible for any losses, direct or indirect, that are incurred as a result of the use of the information contained within this document, including, but not limited to, errors, omissions, or inaccuracies.

Your Free Gift
(only available for a limited time)

Thanks for getting this book! If you want to learn more about various spirituality topics, then join Mari Silva's community and get a free guided meditation MP3 for awakening your third eye. This guided meditation mp3 is designed to open and strengthen ones third eye so you can experience a higher state of consciousness. Simply visit the link below the image to get started.

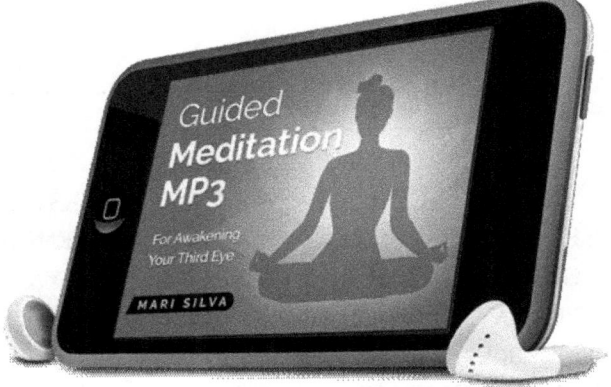

https://spiritualityspot.com/meditation

Or, Scan the QR code!

Table of Contents

PART 1: KRIYA YOGA FOR BEGINNERS...1
   INTRODUCTION 2
   CHAPTER 1: KRIYA YOGA BASICS 4
   CHAPTER 2: YOUR SUBTLE BODY AND THE CHAKRAS 14
   CHAPTER 3: FROM SAMADHI TO KUNDALINI AWAKENING.... 29
   CHAPTER 4: GETTING READY FOR THE PATH OF KRIYA 39
   CHAPTER 5: PRANAYAMA: THE ART OF BREATHING.............. 48
   CHAPTER 6: MUDRAS AND MANTRAS 58
   CHAPTER 7: KRIYA MEDITATION TECHNIQUES 68
   CHAPTER 8: ASANAS: KRIYA POSES TO MASTER 78
   CHAPTER 9: KRIYA YOGA SEQUENCES: PUTTING IT ALL TOGETHER 89
   CHAPTER 10: YOUR DAILY KRIYA PRACTICE 101
   CONCLUSION 108
PART 2: TURIYA 110
   INTRODUCTION 111
   CHAPTER 1: WHAT IS TURIYA, OR PURE CONSCIOUSNESS?... 113
   CHAPTER 2: HINDU PHILOSOPHY BASICS 124
   CHAPTER 3: SHAKTI AND SHIVA, A DIVINE UNION 134
   CHAPTER 4: SAMADHI: THE PURPOSE OF MEDITATION AND YOGA 144
   CHAPTER 5: YOGA POSES THAT PAVE THE WAY TO TURIYA 154
   CHAPTER 6: USING PRANAYAMA TO INDUCE TURIYA 173

- CHAPTER 7: MEDITATION TECHNIQUES TO TRY NOW 184
- CHAPTER 8: USEFUL MANTRAS AND MUDRAS 193
- CHAPTER 9: YOGA SEQUENCES TO UNLOCK TURIYA 201
- CHAPTER 10: YOUR DAILY STEPS TOWARDS TURIYA 210
- CONCLUSION 216
- HERE'S ANOTHER BOOK BY MARI SILVA THAT YOU MIGHT LIKE 218
- YOUR FREE GIFT (ONLY AVAILABLE FOR A LIMITED TIME) 219
- REFERENCES 220

Part 1: Kriya Yoga for Beginners

The Ultimate Guide to Yoga Asanas, Mudras, Meditation, Pranayama, Kundalini Awakening, and Samadhi

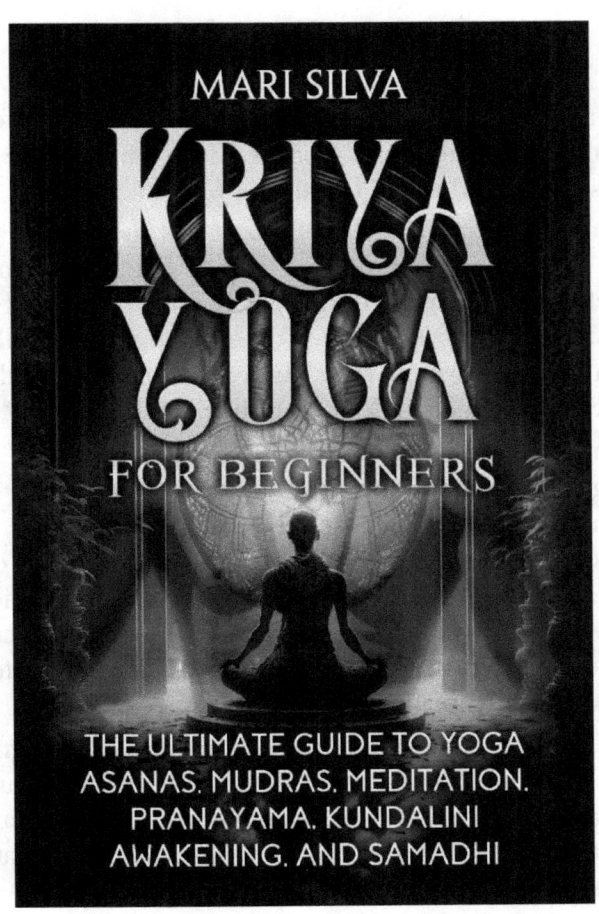

Introduction

Have you ever wanted to experience true inner peace? To feel a sense of oneness with the Universe? Kriya Yoga is an ancient practice that can help you reach these goals and much more.

Kriya Yoga is a unique style of yoga that has been practiced for centuries by yogis and spiritual seekers. This powerful system of techniques helps you still your mind, purify your body, and expand your consciousness. Its goal is to help you understand yourself deeply and connect with the divine within you. The extent of peace and stillness that can be achieved through Kriya Yoga is unlike anything else.

In Hinduism, the term "kriya" means "action," "effort," or "service." So, Kriya Yoga can be translated to the "yoga of action" or the "yoga of effort." This name is fitting because Kriya Yoga is a practice that requires effort and dedication. At its core, Kriya Yoga relies on breathing techniques that guide your breath up and down through different regions of your body. These techniques strengthen your lungs, increase oxygen supply, clear toxins from the blood, and naturally build greater health and vitality in all aspects of your being.

In addition, Kriya Yoga includes various postures that align the physical body with breath to encourage good energy flow throughout your body. Meditation practices such as mantra repetition and silent witnessing encourage you to quiet your thoughts to better find inner peace and a true connection with the divine spark within you. The goal of Kriya Yoga is not simply to achieve physical health or mental peace but rather to reach a state of spiritual awakening and self-realization.

This comprehensive guide will find all the information you need to get started with Kriya Yoga. We will begin by exploring the basics of this ancient practice and discussing its goals. From its history and origins to the different techniques that make up this system, you'll gain a thorough understanding of Kriya Yoga. Then, we will move on to more specific techniques, including instructions for different breathing exercises, postures, and meditation practices.

We will then move on to preparing your body and mind for a daily Kriya Yoga practice. This will involve discussing the importance of setting an intention, finding a comfortable place to practice, and setting aside time for your practice each day. We will also explore the different benefits that you can experience from a Kriya Yoga session. By the end of this book, you'll have everything you need to incorporate Kriya Yoga into your daily life and begin your journey of self-discovery and inner peace.

Most people new to yoga find that they need guidance when getting started. That's why we've put together this comprehensive guide to Kriya Yoga. The benefits of this practice are vast, and we hope this book will help you experience them for yourself. So, if you are looking for a powerful way to still your mind, purify your body, and connect with something more splendid, Kriya Yoga may be just what you need. With regular practice, this ancient practice can truly transform your life and help you achieve deeper states of awareness where healing, wisdom, love, and true happiness await!

Chapter 1: Kriya Yoga Basics

Kriya Yoga is a type of Yoga that has been practiced in India for centuries. This form of Yoga is considered one of the "active" types, as it emphasizes physical movements and postures. However, what truly sets Kriya Yoga apart from other kinds of Yoga is its focus on spiritual development. Many people use kriya as a tool to accelerate their spiritual progress and reach higher levels of consciousness more quickly.

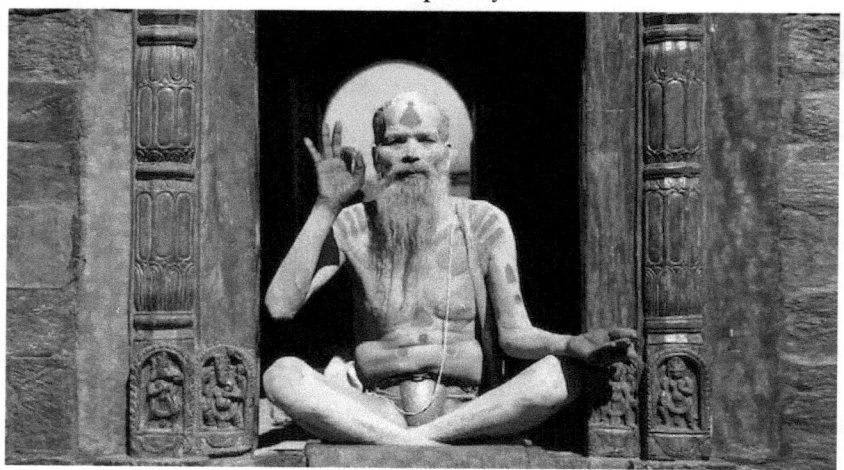

Kriya yoga has been practiced in India for centuries.
https://unsplash.com/photos/-8ZESyFapTk

This chapter will explore the history of Kriya Yoga, what makes it different from other types, and the many benefits that it can offer, both spiritually and physically. We will also take a closer look at the five main branches of Kriya Yoga. Whether you are a seasoned yogi or someone exploring the practice for the first time, Kriya Yoga can help deepen your connection with yourself and make meaningful progress on your journey toward enlightenment.

A Tool for Spiritual Seekers

Kriya Yoga is a powerful system of meditation used by spiritual seekers for centuries. This ancient practice harnesses the power of breath and concentration to create a deep state of inner stillness. For those new to Kriya Yoga, the key is to start with simple breathing exercises that gradually build up toward the more advanced techniques. These exercises can be performed individually or in a group setting and require total focus and commitment to be truly effective. Although it may take time and effort to master, this discipline ultimately provides a powerful framework for achieving spiritual growth and liberation from suffering. If you are looking for a tool for your spiritual journey, the benefits will amaze you!

The Active Aspect of Yoga

At its core, Yoga is a practice that promotes physical, mental, and spiritual wellbeing. In Kriya Yoga, various postures and movements are combined with specific breathing techniques to circulate energy through the body and cultivate deep states of meditative awareness. Unlike other types of Yoga that focus on gentle stretching and relaxation, Kriya Yoga requires a great deal of concentration and personal discipline. Engaging both mind and body helps practitioners develop mental clarity and improved physical health. Whether you want to deepen your meditation practice or increase your fitness levels, Kriya Yoga has something to offer everyone.

History of Kriya Yoga

Kriya Yoga has been around for thousands of years. Originating in ancient India, it was first introduced in a text known as the Yoga Sutras of Patanjali, which outlined various aspects of this profound meditation technique. Over time, Kriya Yoga became popular among spiritual seekers from all backgrounds, and it soon spread worldwide.

One of the unique features of Kriya Yoga is the emphasis on breathwork. Through deep and conscious breathing, practitioners tap into the innermost parts of their consciousness, dissolving barriers and bringing about profound transformations at both a physical and spiritual level. In addition, Kriya Yoga includes other elements such as physical postures, body locks called bandhas, visualization techniques called tratakas, and focused concentration exercises called pranayamas that can help regulate one's energy flow.

Today, many different schools of Kriya Yoga teach various methods and styles. Whether you are embarking on an intensive course or simply looking for inspiration in your daily meditation practice, Kriya Yoga offers a rich array of tools to support you on your journey toward enlightenment.

What Makes Kriya Yoga Different?

Kriya Yoga is an ancient form of meditation that offers many unique benefits to practitioners of this discipline. Unlike other types of Yoga, Kriya focuses primarily on breath and movement, encouraging a tangible approach to mindfulness. At the same time, Kriya also emphasizes the development of inner qualities like peace, compassion, and clarity. Many people find that these qualities are enhanced by the practice of Kriya and can help them live more fulfilling lives. In addition, Kriya incorporates a range of supplementary practices like chanting and affirmations that further strengthen the mind-body connection and help practitioners tap into their full potential. Suppose you're looking for a highly effective form of meditation that goes beyond the typical experience. In that case, Kriya Yoga may be just what you've been searching for.

Spiritual Benefits of Kriya Yoga

Kriya Yoga has been used for thousands of years to enhance mental clarity, focus, and inner peace. At its core, it involves prolonged periods of intense meditation and deep breathing exercises. These practices help calm the mind and center one's thoughts on deeper truths and higher ideals. In addition, Kriya Yoga can positively impact mental health, improving symptoms of depression and anxiety in many people who practice it regularly. Furthermore, this ancient practice can also strengthen relationships by helping individuals to see others with compassion and understanding rather than judgment or negativity. Kriya Yoga offers many spiritual benefits that are well worth exploring for anyone looking to connect more deeply with themselves or others.

1. Spiritual Awakening

Kriya Yoga promotes a deep and meaningful spiritual awakening. This ancient form of Yoga incorporates a host of meditation techniques and breathing exercises, all aimed at helping the practitioner align their mind, body, and soul. By doing so, Kriya Yoga can facilitate a profound state of inner peace, helping us to tune into our highest potential. Additionally, this practice promotes feelings of connection with others and with the universe as a whole. Overall, the benefits of Kriya Yoga are many and far-reaching, making it an essential tool for anyone seeking a deeper sense of spiritual wellbeing. Whether we meditate alone or in groups, Kriya Yoga invites us on a journey toward greater understanding, self-love, and compassion for all beings. When we become fully aware of our true nature, our bodies get rejuvenated and become full of energy - a sign that our moment of true spiritual awakening has arrived!

2. Improved Meditation Practices

Kriya Yoga can also help improve our regular meditation practices. By incorporating a variety of breathing exercises and focused concentration techniques, Kriya helps us still the mind and connect with our deepest truths. In addition, Kriya's emphasis on the body-mind connection can also help us develop a more embodied approach to meditation. As we become more attuned to our physical sensations, we can begin to let go of any mental clutter or distractions that may be preventing us from truly sinking into our meditation practice. For many people, Kriya Yoga is a gateway into more profound states of meditation.

3. Enhanced Mindfulness

Kriya Yoga can also enhance our mindfulness practices. This form of Yoga emphasizes the significance of being present in each and every moment without judgment or attachment. By encouraging us to focus on our breath and bodily sensations, Kriya Yoga helps us to ground ourselves in the here and now. Additionally, Kriya's focus on compassion and understanding can help us see others more clearly and kindly. Through the practice of Kriya Yoga, we can learn to approach each moment with fresh eyes, an open heart, and a beginner's mind.

4. Greater Self-Awareness

Kriya Yoga also leads to greater self-awareness. As we become more attuned to our bodily sensations and breath, we can't help but notice any tightness or tension that may be present in our bodies. Additionally, its focus on the present moment can help us become more aware of our thoughts and emotions as they arise. By learning to observe our inner experiences without judgment, we can develop a greater understanding of ourselves and our patterns. With time, we can even learn to use Kriya Yoga as a tool for self-transformation, letting go of any negative thoughts or behaviors that no longer serve us.

5. Heightened Clarity and Intuition

Kriya Yoga heightens our clarity and intuition. This form of Yoga encourages us to trust our intuition and inner voice, which is often a sign of our highest potential. Additionally, Kriya's focus on meditation can help us develop a greater awareness of the subtler aspects of life. As we become more attuned to our breath and bodily sensations, we can also begin to pick up on subtle changes in our environment and the people around us. With time, we may even find that we can sense the future or connect with our loved ones who have passed on.

6. Increased Ability to Manifest Desires

Kriya Yoga can also help us manifest our desires. This form of Yoga teaches us to focus on our intention rather than our outcome. By focusing on what we want to create in our lives, we can better align ourselves with the flow of universal energy. Additionally, Kriya's emphasis on gratitude and compassion can help us to attract more positive energy into our lives. As we learn to let go of attachment and resistance, we can open ourselves up to limitless possibilities.

7. Improved Health and Vitality

Kriya Yoga also leads to improved health and vitality. This form of Yoga helps us release any tension or blockages that may be present in our bodies. Additionally, its focus on breathing and meditation can improve our circulation and respiratory functions. As we learn to take control of our breath, we can also begin to regulate our stress levels and nervous system. With time, we may even find that we have more energy, stamina, and a greater sense of overall wellbeing.

8. Deeper Connection to the Divine

Kriya Yoga helps us develop a deeper connection to the divine. This form of Yoga emphasizes our oneness with all of creation. By focusing on our breath and bodily sensations, we can begin to see the interconnectedness of all life. Kriya's focus on compassion and forgiveness can help us develop a more loving relationship with ourselves and others. As we learn to let go of judgment and fear, we can open ourselves up to a deeper sense of connection with the universe. Through the practice of Kriya Yoga, we can learn to appreciate the sacredness of life itself.

9. Greater Sense of Purpose

Kriya Yoga can also help us find a greater sense of purpose. This form of Yoga encourages us to live in alignment with our highest values. We can better connect with our true nature by focusing on our breath and bodily sensations. Kriya's focus on the present moment can also help us let go of any attachments or preconceptions that we may have about who we are. As we learn to connect with our authentic selves, we can begin to live more authentically. In doing so, we can discover a greater sense of purpose and meaning in our lives.

10. Greater Sense of Peace and Calm

Kriya Yoga involves a process of deep breathing and concentrated focus, which allows you to become deeply rooted in the present moment and free your mind from distractions. It requires mental discipline and active engagement in your inner journey, helping you to connect more deeply with your subconscious thoughts and emotions. Regular practice of this ancient eastern discipline will make you more attuned to the energy within and around you, allowing you to live your life with greater presence, awareness, and joy. Kriya Yoga may be the perfect path for you if you are looking for a way to nourish your soul and deepen your connection with the universe.

Medical Benefits of Kriya Yoga

Kriya Yoga is an ancient system of physical and mental practices that positively affect health and wellbeing. These include improved cardiovascular function, reduced blood pressure, better sleep and digestion, and strengthened immunity. Additionally, it can serve as a natural stress reliever, helping individuals relax and be more present. Overall, this practice can support physical and emotional wellbeing, making it a valuable tool for anyone looking to achieve greater health and wellness. Whether you're looking to increase your energy levels or simply experience greater peace of mind, Kriya Yoga may be the perfect solution for you!

1. Lower Blood Pressure

Research by the University of Texas Southwestern Medical Center found that Kriya Yoga can help lower blood pressure. The study participants who took part in the Kriya Yoga intervention showed significant reductions in both systolic and diastolic blood pressure. Additionally, the Kriya Yoga group also had greater improvements in heart rate and respiratory function. Reducing stress levels can decrease blood pressure, as high stress levels are known to contribute to hypertension. Additionally, by stretching and strengthening the body through various postures, Kriya Yoga can improve overall cardiovascular function and circulation.

2. More Balanced Hormones

Anyone who has experienced the ups and downs of hormone imbalances can attest that maintaining healthy hormone levels is crucial for our overall wellbeing. Whether your hormones are out of whack due to a medical condition like PCOS or simply because you're experiencing the effects of menopause, keeping your hormones balanced can be essential for combating tiredness, mood swings, and other common symptoms associated with hormonal fluctuations. How do you maintain more balanced hormone levels? According to recent research, practicing Kriya Yoga may be an effective way to achieve that.

In a study published in 2015, researchers at the University of Rajasthan found that Kriya Yoga can help improve hormone levels in postmenopausal women. The study found that women who practiced it regularly tended to have lower testosterone levels and better insulin sensitivity than those who did not. In addition, women who regularly engaged in Kriya Yoga also reported feeling less stressed and more relaxed than those who did not. These findings suggest that regular Kriya practices could help naturally rebalance our hormones by improving insulin sensitivity, reducing stress levels, and promoting relaxation.

3. Improved Digestion

As anyone who has experienced digestive issues can attest, improved digestion is one of the biggest benefits of practicing Kriya Yoga. Several physical mechanisms can explain this effect. First, Kriya Yoga is known for activating and cleansing the digestive system, allowing it to function more efficiently. This, in turn, can reduce symptoms such as bloating, constipation, and gas. Additionally, regular practice can help calm the nervous system and reduce muscle tension throughout the body. This combination reduces stress levels and thus improves digestion and relieves chronic pain that may be linked to irregular digestion and bowel movement. If you're looking to improve your digestion or relieve your digestive problems, consider incorporating some form of Kriya Yoga into your routine!

Branching Out: The Five Branches of Kriya Yoga

There are five main branches of Kriya Yoga, each with its unique focus and benefits. The five branches are:

1. Kriya Kundalini Pranayama

This branch of Kriya Yoga focuses on the breath, specifically on regulating and controlling the breath. Kriya Kundalini Pranayama is a powerful technique that harnesses the energies of the body and mind to promote healing and wellness. This breathing practice has a variety of benefits, including reduced stress and anxiety, improved circulation, and enhanced energy levels. Additionally, the energy center located at the base of the spine is activated during Kriya Kundalini Pranayama, allowing users to connect more easily with their intuition and experience heightened creativity.

2. Kriya Dhyana Yoga

This branch is a unique form of Yoga that combines physical postures, breath work, and meditation techniques to achieve physical, mental, and spiritual balance. Unlike other types of Yoga, which emphasize one aspect or another, Kriya Dhyana simultaneously encompasses all three aspects of Yoga. Practicing this holistic Yoga style can awaken your body's connection to spirit and experience deep relaxation and inner calm. Whether you are new to this world or a seasoned practitioner, Kriya Dhyana can help you achieve greater harmony in both your body and mind.

3. Kriya Mantra Yoga

Kriya Mantra Yoga is a powerful and transformative system of Yoga that harnesses the power of mantras, or sacred sound vibrations, to help practitioners experience deep physical, mental, and spiritual awakenings. The kriyas, or cleansing practices that make up this Yoga practice, also work to purify the body by toning and activating various energy centers along the spine. With regular practice of Kriya Mantra Yoga, one can unlock a whole new level of inner peace and wisdom that goes far beyond simple physical health and fitness. If you're looking to experience true transformation in your life, then look no further than Kriya Mantra Yoga. With a little practice every day, you can unleash your highest health and happiness potential!

4. Kriya Bhakti Yoga

Kriya Bhakti Yoga is an ancient practice that has been gaining popularity in recent years as more and more people look for alternative ways to enhance their physical, mental, and spiritual wellbeing. At its core, Kriya Bhakti Yoga is all about devoting one's time, energy, and attention to improving oneself and one's community. This can be accomplished through various techniques, including focused breathing exercises, meditation practices, mantras, and visualization techniques. By focusing on our connection with the universe and cultivating positive thought patterns, we can work to cultivate our inner potential and achieve greater happiness and harmony within ourselves and in our relationships with others. No matter what your goals are, Kriya Bhakti offers something for everyone.

5. Kriya Jnana Yoga

Kriya Jnana Yoga is a branch of Yoga that focuses on the mind and intuition as keys to unlocking spiritual awareness and enlightenment. This practice centers on mindfulness meditation, a deep concentration technique that allows practitioners to go beyond their surface-level thoughts and feelings and tap into the power of their intuition. By opening themselves up to this intuitive wisdom, Kriya Jnana Yogis believe they can truly connect with their inner selves and come to a deeper understanding of their world. Whether seeking greater personal growth or gaining insight into their place in the universe, Kriya Jnana Yoga helps practitioners at all stages of their journey toward self-realization.

Kriya Yoga is a spiritual practice that involves focusing on one's inner self while performing certain mental and physical exercises. Today, it is practiced by millions worldwide as a tool for achieving inner peace and outer harmony. But how did Kriya Yoga originate, and what makes this ancient practice so fascinating?

Some historians believe that Kriya Yoga was first developed in India over two thousand years ago. According to these accounts, the practice was mastered by an Indian sage named Patanjali, who used it to control his breath and remain focused at all times. After many generations of careful cultivation and refinement, it eventually spread from India to other cultures throughout the world.

Today, many people enjoy exploring the rich history and unique philosophy of Kriya Yoga. Whether you are interested in meditation, self-discovery, or simply looking to try something new and exciting, this ancient practice has much to offer. With its focus on achieving greater balance in mind and body, it can be life-changing for those who fully commit to it. If you're looking for a deeper connection with your inner self or a path toward personal enlightenment, perhaps it's time to try Kriya Yoga!

Chapter 2: Your Subtle Body and the Chakras

The subtle body in the Sanskrit language is called "Sukshma Sharira." "Sukshma" is translated to subtle, and "Sharira" is translated to the body. The subtle body, or the astral body as it is often called, consists of the ego, the intellect, and the mind. The physical body needs the subtle body to function properly since it's the one that supplies it with the energy it needs to survive. Hindu philosophy believes that each person is divided into three bodies:

- The subtle body
- The gross physical body
- The causal body

According to yogis and their philosophy, these three bodies make up each person's consciousness. It is the energy of the subtle body that connects the other two bodies together. Most people are only concerned with the physical body, but the subtle body is of equal significance. It consists of several energy layers necessary for your body to maintain its vitality. These different layers of energy vibrate at various frequencies that increase with each layer. However, unlike the physical body and all its vital organs, the subtle body is invisible as it is something beyond what is physical. You can still feel the subtle body by awakening your third eye, which is similar to the sixth sense.

The energy flowing through your subtle body is prana, life energy, or chi. The three words have the same meanings but in different languages.

Prana is a Sanskrit word, and Chi is a Chinese word, and both mean life energy and life force energy. Prana refers to the universal energy that flows through all living beings. This vital energy is never stagnant but must always be moving through the body. When prana stops flowing or gets blocked, this can impact your physical, mental, and emotional health. Balanced prana will have a positive impact on every aspect of your life. This energy is responsible for all your vital physical functions, like healing, digestion, and breathing.

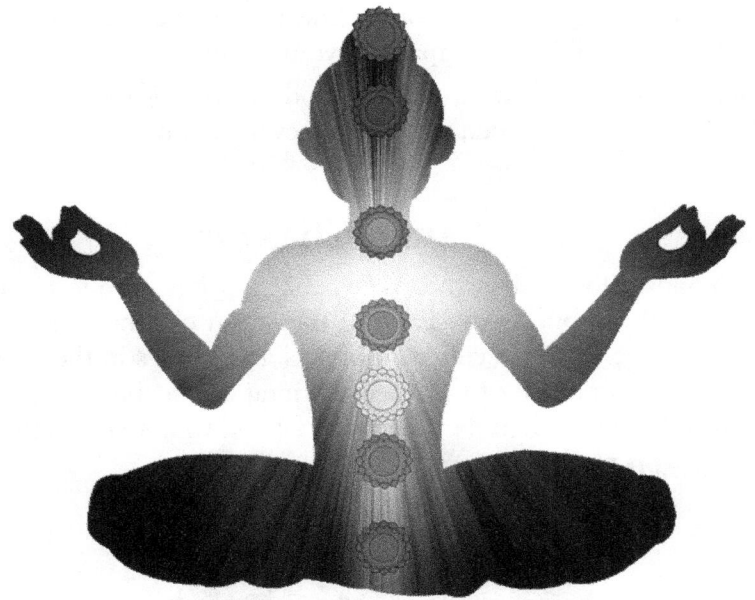

The energy that flows through your body is called Prana.
https://pixabay.com/es/illustrations/yoga-chakras-s%c3%admbolo-buda-6513344/

Prana must be distributed throughout every part of your physical body. This happens through specific channels called the nadis. The nadis don't exist in the physical body. They exist in the subtle body. Although there are thousands of nadis, there are three main ones:

- Sushumna
- Ida
- Pingala

The three nadis begin at the spine's base and end at the head. The Pingala and the Ida intersect with one another and connect opposite the nostrils. The Sushumna nadis travels from the spine upwards until it reaches the head. The point of intersection between the Sushumna and the Ida and Pingala is the location of the seven chakras. The thousands of nadis connect with the seven chakras. The chakras distribute the life energy/prana to every organ and cell in the body.

Think of the nadis as a network that carries the energy in your body. They bring energy to the chakras, which distribute it to the body. The nadis are as vital as the arteries and the veins and have the same purpose. What would happen to your body if any of your arteries were blocked? This will restrict the blood flow, resulting in serious health issues. The same can happen when the nadis or chakras are blocked. The energy flow is restricted, and you'll feel its impact on your health.

Keeping the energy flowing in your body is vital for your wellbeing. However, this can only happen when your seven chakras are balanced and opened.

The Seven Chakras

Chakra is a Sanskrit word that means "wheel," but it is used to refer to the focal points of the subtle body. Each of the seven chakras is responsible for distributing energy to specific vital organs and nerves in the body. It is essential for your wellbeing to learn everything about the seven chakras, including how to know when they are blocked and what to do in that case.

Root Chakra (Muladhara)

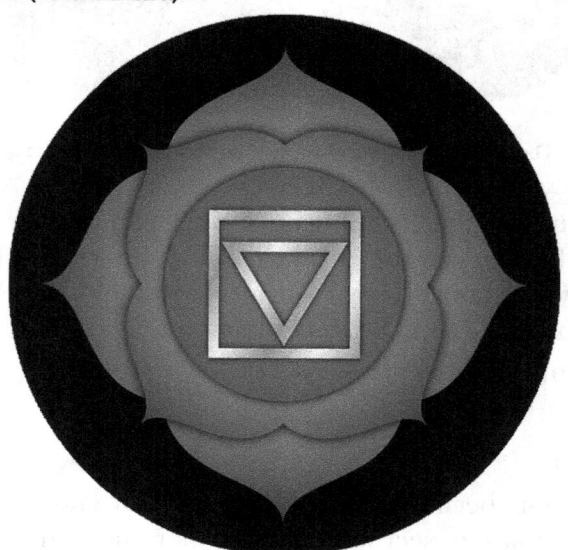

Root Chakra.
https://pixabay.com/es/illustrations/ra%c3%adz-chakra-energ%c3%ada-chi-espiritual-2533091/

The root chakra is the first of the seven chakras; therefore, it acts as the base of the body. It is responsible for all the vital functions necessary to keep you alive, like sleeping and breathing, and it keeps you grounded. It also provides you with a sense of security.

Color

Red

Mantra

Lam

Element

Earth

Stone/Crystal

Hematite and red jasper

Yoga Pose to Unblock It

Mountain pose

Location

At the base of the spine

Correspondences

Food, money, and anything related to your survival

Blocked Root Chakra Symptoms

You'll feel the impact of a blocked root chakra on your mental health as you begin experiencing nightmares, anxiety, and unexplained fears resulting from a sense of insecurity. Frustration and emotional instability are also symptoms of a blocked root chakra. You'll also feel lost as you struggle to find your purpose in life. Your physical health will suffer as you experience pain in different body parts, like your feet, lower back, and legs. Any imbalance in this chakra can also affect your bladder and colon.

An overactive root chakra can make you indulge in unhealthy behaviors like overeating and having too much sex.

Open Root Chakra Symptoms

You'll feel grounded, strong, and energetic when the root chakra is open. Your digestion will also improve. You'll feel more independent and committed in your relationships and career. The negative emotions you experienced when this chakra was blocked will be replaced with positive ones like stability, strength, confidence, and balance. You'll feel strong and able to stand up for yourself and withstand whatever life throws at you.

Unblocking the Root Chakra

Yoga is one of the best methods to help you unblock all your chakras. The best poses for the root chakras include the Malasana, Warrior I, and the Balasana. These poses will help ground you and bring the root chakra back to balance. You can also carry healing stones or crystals associated with the root chakra or meditate with them, like red jasper, obsidian, and ruby. Incorporating certain types of food, like peppers, onions, tomatoes, carrots, parsnips, strawberries, and beets, into your diet will also do the trick.

Sacral Chakra (Swadhisthana)

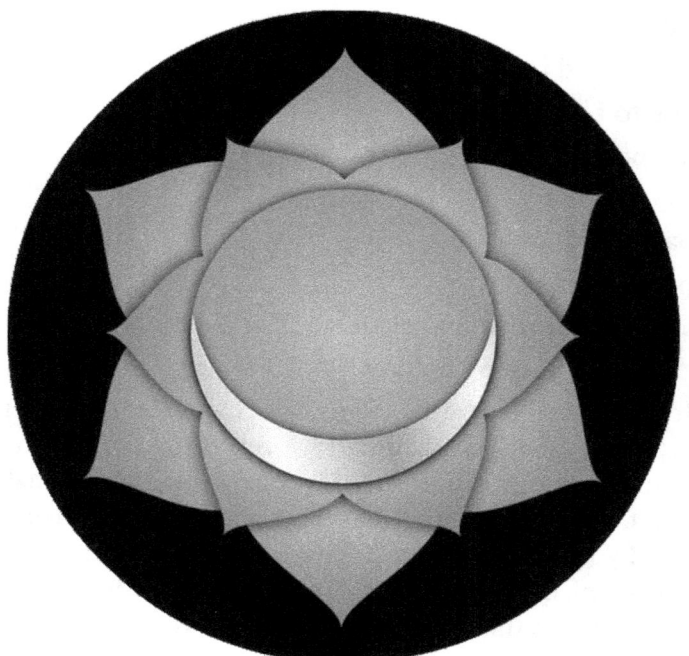

Sacral Chakra.
https://pixabay.com/es/illustrations/sacro-chakra-energ%c3%ada-chi-2533094/

The sacral chakra is associated with sexuality, self-esteem, and creativity. This chakra helps you better understand your emotions and make sense of what you are feeling. It opens your senses, so you can also understand what people are feeling. This chakra governs all your feelings and emotions, like pleasures and passions. Think of any emotion that brings you happiness; the sacral chakra is most likely behind them.

Color

Orange

Mantra

Vam

Element

Water

Stone/Crystal

Sunstone, carnelian, and tiger's eye

Yoga Pose to Unblock It

Goddess pose

Location

Pelvic area in the lower abdomen

Correspondences

Wellbeing, sexuality, and pleasure

Blocked Sacral Chakra Symptoms

When the sacral chakra is blocked, you'll experience an imbalance in your emotions that will manifest in explosive anger and irritability. You'll also become consumed with sexual and manipulative thoughts. Lack of creativity and energy are also symptoms of a blocked sacral chakra. You'll feel uninspired and depressed and may struggle with addiction problems. More often than not, you'll feel that your life is out of control. Your sexuality will also take a toll as you may suffer from hormonal problems or low libido. When this chakra is blocked, it can also affect your physical health, as you'll suffer from digestion issues, pain in your pelvis, menstrual problems, exhaustion, and immunity problems.

An overactive sacral chakra will result in out-of-control behavior associated with addiction or sex. Your emotions will also be unstable and will fluctuate between extreme highs and lows.

Open Sacral Chakra Symptoms

Think of a happy person walking down the street with a big smile and a positive and welcoming attitude. This is what it looks like to have an open sacral chakra. It makes you friendly, warm, joyful, and passionate. You'll also enjoy everything life has to offer in moderation without over-indulgence.

Unblocking the Sacral Chakra

You can try yoga poses like Mandukasana, Bhujangasana, and Kapotasana. Placing healing crystals on your pelvic area while meditating or bathing can help open your sacral chakra. Orange crystals are your best option here since it's the color of this chakra. You can try crystals like orange calcite, carnelian, and garnet. Incorporating these foods into your diet can help balance your sacral chakra (like mango, honey, pumpkin, and oranges).

Solar Plexus Chakra (Manipura)

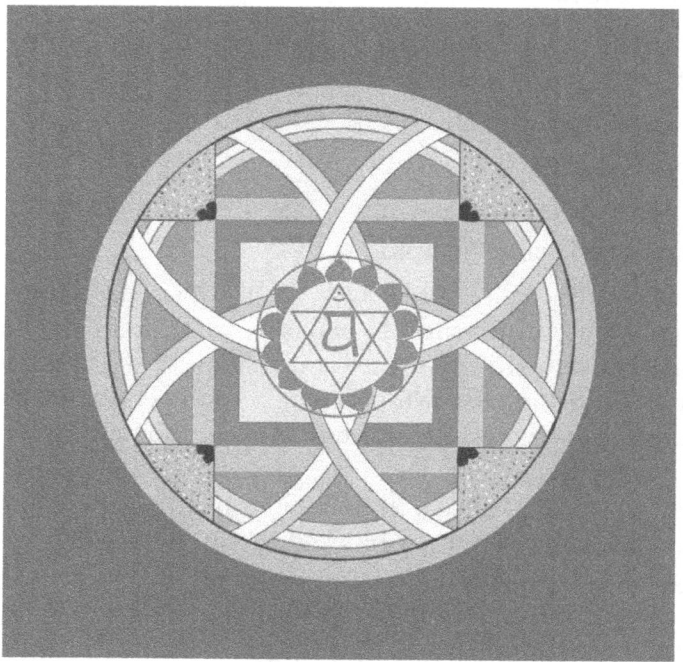

Sacral Chakra.
https://creazilla.com/nodes/1663672-chakra-mandala-meditation-illustration

This chakra is associated with confidence and the ability to remain in control. It governs your self-esteem and gives you a sense of individualism and personal power. It is the most powerful of the seven chakras. It encourages you to be brave, stand up for yourself, and set healthy boundaries.

Color

Yellow

Mantra

Ram

Element

Fire

Stone/Crystal

Amber and pyrite

Yoga Pose to Unblock It

Boat pose

Location

The stomach area

Correspondences

Self-esteem and self-confidence

Blocked Solar Plexus Chakra Symptoms

The emotions associated with this blocked chakra are aggression, ego, and anger. You may also experience health issues in some vital organs, like the liver. Some people also suffer from diabetes, digestive issues, and stomach issues. Emotional symptoms are also common when this chakra is blocked, like anger issues, depression, and self-esteem issues. You may also experience feelings of self-doubt and shame. A blocked solar plexus chakra can make you indecisive and struggle with remaining in control, whether of your temper or your life in general. You'll constantly feel down as a result of your self-esteem issues. Consequently, you'll start acting on these feelings. You'll procrastinate your work, be apathetic, and will be an easy target for people to take advantage of you.

When this chakra is overactive, you'll act maniacally and become hyperactive and power-hungry.

Open Solar Plexus Chakra Symptoms

When this chakra is balanced, you'll feel more focused, energetic, and productive, and your self-esteem will improve. You'll have the confidence to be who you are and express yourself freely with no fear or hesitation.

Unblocking the Solar Plexus Chakra

Yoga poses like Navasana, Virabhadrasana, and Dhanurasana can help unblock the solar plexus chakra. Meditating with yellow crystals or placing them on your stomach area is also helpful. You can use crystals like yellow quartz, citrine, and yellow calcite. Adding yellow food to your diet, like bananas, yellow peppers, and pineapple can bring the solar plexus chakra back to balance.

Heart Chakra (Anahata)

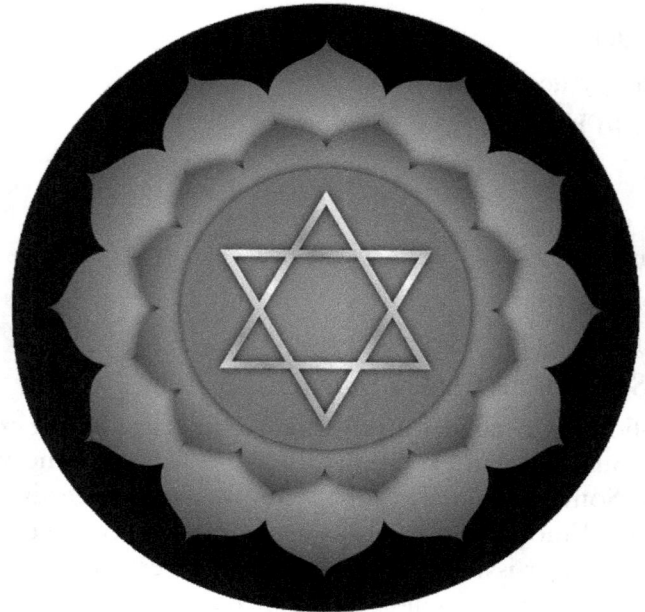

Heart Chakra.
https://www.needpix.com/photo/1027035/heart-chakra-energy-chi

This is the heart chakra, which governs all matters of the heart, like love, romance, and relationships. It is associated with emotions like passion, compassion, and attachment. Love is the keyword here, as the heart chakra allows you to love, accept love, and love yourself. It is the fourth chakra which means that it stands in a unique position in the middle of the seven chakras.

Color
Green and pink

Mantra
Yam

Element
Air

Stone/Crystal
Malachite, jade, rose quartz

Yoga Pose to Unblock It
Camel pose

Location
Around the heart area

Correspondences
Inner peace, love, and joy

Blocked Heart Chakra Symptoms

When the heart chakra is blocked, this will naturally impact your emotions. You'll feel anxious, moody, afraid, angry, and jealous. You will not be able to trust the people in your life. A closed heart chakra will make you struggle to open up to anyone, even your family and friends. You'll struggle with trust issues and will live in fear that those close to you may betray you. Your relationships will suffer as you struggle with giving and receiving love. You will not be able to forgive, forget, or move on from the past.

An overactive heart chakra can make you too attached to your loved ones . . . needy, possessive, and dependent on them.

Open Heart Chakra Symptoms

An open heart chakra will make you a caring, compassionate, friendly, motivated, and optimistic individual. You'll experience empathy and be able to feel and relate to what other people are feeling. It gives you the ability to forgive others and awakens your spirit. You'll radiate positive vibes and give and receive love easily.

Unblocking the Heart Chakra

Practice yoga poses like Garudasana and Ustrasana to unblock the heart chakra. Wear necklaces with crystals associated with the heart chakra, like jade, emerald, and watermelon tourmaline. Green vegetables can also heal the heart chakra.

Throat Chakra (Vishuddha)

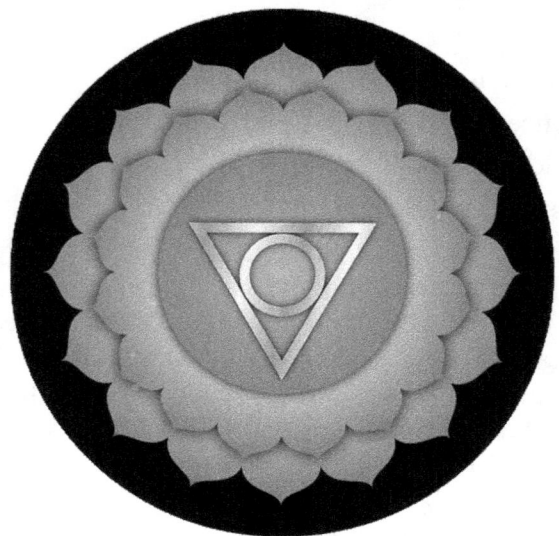

Throat chakra.
https://pixabay.com/es/illustrations/garganta-chakra-chi-energ%c3%ada-2533108/

As the throat chakra, it is responsible for your ability to communicate and express yourself. It's the chakra that gives your voice power so you can confidently speak your truth.

Color
Blue
Mantra
Ham
Element
Space
Stone/Crystal
Aquamarine
Yoga Pose to Unblock It
Fish pose
Location
The throat area
Correspondences
Truth, communication, and self-expression

Blocked Throat Chakra Symptoms

When the throat chakra is blocked, you cannot communicate your thoughts. You'll also become unusually quiet and shy and struggle with self-expression. Listening to what others say will feel like a chore since you'll struggle with all types of communication. You'll hide your true self out of fear of being judged. Some physical symptoms may manifest like headaches, sore throats, and tensed shoulders and neck.

An overactive throat chakra will make you dominate the conversation and be judgmental.

Open Throat Chakra Symptoms

An open-throat chakra will allow you to express yourself better and improve your communication skills. You'll also be able to listen intently to what others are communicating to you without misunderstanding. This chakra allows you to stand up for your values and beliefs, as no one will be able to silence your voice.

Unblocking the Throat Chakra

Practice yoga poses like Matsyasana and Halasana to open up your throat chakra. Place blue crystals on your throat (like aquamarine and lapis lazuli) while meditating. Add blue foods to your diet, like blueberries.

Third-Eye Chakra (Ajna)

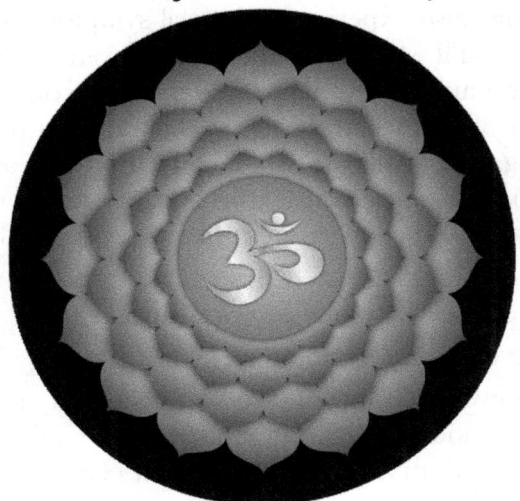

Third eye chakra.
https://www.needpix.com/photo/1027042/crown-chakra-energy-chi

This chakra is associated with self-knowledge, insight, and intelligence. It helps you see the big picture and perceive things on a deeper level without clouded judgment. Your other chakras usually impact this chakra, so if they get imbalanced, so will your third eye chakra.

Color

Indigo

Mantra

Om

Element

Light

Stone/Crystal

Amethyst and labradorite

Yoga Pose to Unblock It

Child's pose

Location

The forehead

Correspondences

Wisdom, Intuition, and imagination

Blocked Third Eye Chakra Symptoms

A blocked third eye chakra can make you scared of success and egotistical. You may also experience physical symptoms like blurry vision and headaches. You'll struggle with trusting your own judgment and tapping into your intuition. Feeling disconnected from your intuition is another symptom of a blocked third eye chakra. As a result, you'll over-analyze everything, which will overwhelm and frustrate you. Ignoring your intuition can also make a person live in anxiety and fear. You may also struggle with various health issues like dizziness, headaches, and depression.

An overactive chakra can make you over-imaginative.

Open Third Eye Chakra Symptoms

An open third eye chakra will make you confident and encourage you to tap into your intuition. You'll be attuned to the spiritual and physical world. You'll gain wisdom as you let go of your ego and begin listening to your intuition.

Unblocking the Third Eye Chakra

Meditation and visualization are key factors in helping you open your third eye chakra. Crystals like sugilite, amethyst, and sapphire can also do the job. Stick to purple food like grapes, plums, and eggplants.

Crown Chakra (Sahasrara)

The crown chakra is the last of the seven chakras and is responsible for enlightenment and spirituality. It invites wisdom into your life.

Color
White and violet

Mantra
Aum

Element
None

Stone/Crystal
Clear Quartz

Yoga Pose to Unblock It
Headstand

Location
The top of the head

Correspondences
Spiritual connection and beauty (inner and outer)

Blocked Crown Chakra Symptoms

A closed crown chakra can lead to destructive emotions and extreme sadness. You'll feel disconnected from the world and the people around you. As a result, you'll lose your way and struggle to find a purpose in your life.

When the crown chakra is overactive, you'll forgo the spiritual and become obsessed with acquiring materialistic belongings.

Open Crown Chakra Symptoms

An open crown chakra can help you reach a higher consciousness. However, having an open crown chakra is very rare but not impossible. It can also allow you to connect with others, the divine, and your higher self.

Unblocking the Crown Chakra

Crown Mudra, Baddha, and Padmasana are some of the most effective yoga poses that can help you open your crown chakra. Place purple crystals like diamonds, selenite, and moonstone on your forehead. Fasting for a few hours can also help unblock the crown chakra.

How Kriya Yoga Helps in Awakening and Healing the Chakras

Kriya yoga helps you relax your body and mind. This type of yoga can also stimulate the chakras and purify them. It can also improve your chakras' functions and make them perform optimally. Kriya Yoga cleanses the chakras so the prana can easily flow through them.

Not seeing something doesn't make it any less real. You can't see the subtle body or even feel it, but this doesn't mean that it isn't needed. The subtle body is where the seven chakras exist. They receive the prana and distribute it throughout your body to improve your health and wellbeing. Blocked chakras can have a negative impact on your physical and mental health. Every chakra is associated with a color. Learn these colors, as they will help heal your chakras. Learn the difference between a blocked and an open chakra so you'll realize when something feels off and take the necessary steps. When all your chakras are opened, you will notice a difference in every aspect of your life. Always check on yourself and be aware of your emotions.

Chapter 3: From Samadhi to Kundalini Awakening

In yogic tradition, two major concepts are often spoken about together, although they are quite different. These concepts are kundalini and samadhi. Kundalini refers to an energy that lies dormant at the base of the spine, while samadhi is a state of religious ecstasy or enlightenment. Though they are two different things, kundalini awakening can only be achieved through a state of samadhi. In this chapter, we will first explore kundalini, discussing what it is and how it can be awakened. We will then explore samadhi, discussing the different stages of this state and how it can be achieved. Finally, we will discuss kriyas' role in achieving kundalini awakening and samadhi.

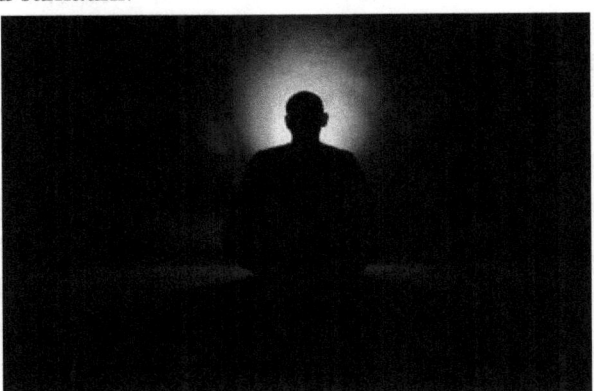

Reaching a state of Kundalini from Samadhi requires focus and practice.
https://pxhere.com/en/photo/1414673

Kundalini

Kundalini is a powerful force that exists at the core of every living being. Some believe that it rests at the base of the spine, dormant and waiting to be awakened. When this energy is unleashed, it rises and travels through the body, connecting with different chakras. The result of this activation is deep healing and spiritual growth. While no one knows exactly how or why kundalini exists, many people have experienced its power firsthand through yoga practices, meditation retreats, or other transformative experiences. Whether you are seeking enlightenment or simply curious about this mysterious force, one thing is clear: kundalini holds great potential for those who are brave enough to tap into it.

A. Kundalini and the Chakras

Kundalini is a term that refers to a type of energy that lies dormant at the base of the spine in most human beings. This force is generally thought to be associated with the account of the "serpent power" described in many ancient mythologies, and it can be awakened through practices like yoga or meditation. Once activated, this energy travels up through the various chakras or energy centers in the body, eventually resulting in deep spiritual awakening and profound changes to one's consciousness.

The seven main chakras are each associated with a different level of consciousness. They are often thought of as steps on a ladder leading up to enlightenment. The first chakra, located at the base of the spine, is known as the Muladhara or "root" chakra. This chakra is associated with the physical body and its needs, such as food, shelter, and safety. The second chakra, located just below the navel, is known as the Svadhisthana or "sacral" chakra. This chakra is associated with pleasure, sexuality, and creativity. The third chakra, located in the solar plexus area, is known as the Manipura or "power" chakra. This chakra is associated with ambition, personal power, and self-esteem.

The fourth chakra, located in the heart area, is known as the Anahata or "unstuck" chakra. This chakra is associated with love, compassion, and forgiveness. The fifth chakra, located in the throat area, is known as the Vishuddha or "clear" chakra. It is associated with communication and self-expression. The sixth chakra, located between the eyebrows, is known as the Ajna or "third eye" chakra. This chakra is associated with intuition, imagination, and wisdom. The seventh chakra, located at the crown of the head, is known as the Sahasrara or "thousand-petaled" chakra. It is associated with spirituality, unity consciousness, and connection to the Divine.

B. The Process of Kundalini Awakening

There are many ways to awaken kundalini energy, and the process can vary depending on the individual. Sometimes, kundalini may be awakened spontaneously through a sudden event or experience, such as a near-death experience, a powerful meditation, or a major life change. For most people, however, kundalini is awakened gradually over time through regular yoga practice, meditation, and other spiritual disciplines.

The process of kundalini awakening can be divided into three main stages:

1. The first stage, known as "prana shakti," is characterized by physical and psychological symptoms such as increased energy levels, anxiety, and irritability. This stage is often associated with a feeling of "restlessness" or "being on edge."
2. The second stage, known as "Chitta shakti," is characterized by mental and emotional symptoms such as racing thoughts, insomnia, and mood swings. This stage is often associated with a feeling of "inner turmoil" or "being pulled in different directions."
3. The third stage, known as "samadhi shakti," is characterized by spiritual symptoms such as a sense of oneness with the universe, profound peace, and bliss. This stage is often associated with a feeling of "enlightenment" or "union with the Divine."

C. What Happens Once Kundalini Is Awakened?

Once kundalini is awakened, it begins to travel up through the chakras, gradually opening and activating each one. This process can take months or even years to complete, often leading to profound changes in consciousness. As kundalini moves through the chakras, we may experience physical, mental, emotional, and spiritual symptoms. These symptoms can be positive and negative and may come and go as kundalini moves through the chakras.

Some of the most common symptoms of kundalini awakening include:
- Increased energy levels
- Changes in sleep patterns
- Changes in appetite

- Intense emotions
- Psychosomatic symptoms
- Paranormal experiences
- Spiritual insights
- Sense of connection to the Divine

As kundalini continues to move up through the chakras, we may also begin to experience more profound changes in consciousness. These changes can include a greater sense of peace and wellbeing, a deeper understanding of the nature of reality, and a stronger connection to the Divine. For some people, kundalini awakening can be a life-changing experience that leads to personal transformation and spiritual growth.

D. How Can Kundalini Awakening be Achieved?

Kundalini awakening can only be achieved through Samadhi. When we reach a state of Samadhi, the kundalini energy can rise through the chakras and awaken our true potential. Once this happens, we may begin to experience the profound changes in consciousness associated with the awakening.

There are many different ways to achieve Samadhi, and the best method will vary from person to person. Some of the most common methods include meditation, yoga, and breath work. Samadhi is not something that can be achieved overnight. It often takes months or even years of dedicated practice to reach this state. However, the rewards of Samadhi are well worth the effort. Once we reach this state, we may begin to experience a sense of oneness with the universe, profound peace, and bliss. We may also find that our lives are transformed in unexpected and wonderful ways.

Samadhi

In the Hindu and Buddhist traditions, Samadhi is a state of deep concentration and oneness with the universe. This high level of awareness can be cultivated through various means, such as meditation, visualization, and mindfulness exercises. As one progresses through these practices and begins to open their mind and heart to the world around them, they may begin to experience moments of Samadhi - the sense of ultimate connection to everything that exists in the universe. Through consistent practice and dedication, we can all tap into this deeper state of being and find peace, contentment, and enlightenment within ourselves. If you want greater spiritual fulfillment or to enhance your overall happiness and wellbeing, dive into Samadhi's world and discover your true self.

A. The Stages of Samadhi

There are three main stages of Samadhi, each with its distinct characteristics.

1. The first stage is known as "samprajnata samadhi" and is characterized by a deep sense of concentration and one-pointedness of mind. This level can be attained through practices such as meditation and mindfulness.
2. The second stage is known as "asamprajnata samadhi" and is characterized by a deep sense of tranquility and bliss. This level can be attained through practices such as mantra repetition and visualization.
3. The third stage is known as "nirvikalpa samadhi" and is characterized by a deep sense of unity with the universe. This level can be attained through practices such as prayer and service to others.

B. Who Can Attain Samadhi?

Anyone can attain samadhi, regardless of their religious beliefs or spiritual practices. All that is required is a willingness to let go of the ego self and open up to the greater reality that exists all around us. Through regular practice and dedicated effort, we can all reach this higher state of consciousness and find true peace and happiness within ourselves. However, it should be noted that the journey to Samadhi is not always easy. There will be times when we feel lost and confused, and there may even be moments when we want to give up entirely. However, if we can persevere through these difficult times, we will eventually reach the end of our journey and the ultimate goal of Samadhi.

C. What Are the Benefits of Samadhi?

There are many benefits to be gained from attaining Samadhi, such as:
- A deeper understanding of the nature of reality
- A stronger connection to the Divine
- A sense of peace and wellbeing
- Enhanced creativity and intuition
- Improved mental and physical health
- Greater clarity of mind

- Increased focus and concentration
- A deeper sense of connection to others
- An overall feeling of happiness and contentment

Suppose you are seeking greater spiritual fulfillment or wish to enhance your overall wellbeing. In that case, Samadhi is something you should explore. You can tap into this deeper state of consciousness through regular practice and find true peace and happiness within yourself.

D. How Is Samadhi Achieved?

There are many ways to achieve Samadhi, but meditation is the most common method. Meditation allows us to still the mind and let go of all the thoughts and worries that constantly fill our heads. As we quiet our minds, we become more aware of the present moment and the beauty that exists all around us. We may also begin to notice the subtle energies that flow through our bodies and connect us to all of life. With regular practice, we can learn to quiet our minds more and more until we eventually reach a state of complete inner peace. Other methods of achieving Samadhi include mantra repetition, visualization, and prayer.

E. What Does Samadhi Feel Like?

When we reach a state of Samadhi, we may feel a deep sense of peace and wellbeing. We may also feel a strong connection to the Divine and a sense of unity with all of life. Some people have even described it as feeling like they are "in love with the world." The renowned mystic Ramana Maharshi once said, "in Samadhi, the 'I' dies, and the Self is revealed." In other words, we let go of our ego selves and become one with the greater reality. This can be a very profoundly moving experience that completely changes our lives.

F. What Happens After Samadhi?

After reaching a state of Samadhi, we may find that our lives are completely transformed. We may see the world in a new way and feel a deeper sense of connection to all of life. We may also develop new abilities, such as enhanced creativity and intuition. In addition, our mental and physical health may improve, and we may even find that we can manifest our desires more easily. However, remember that Samadhi is not a goal to be attained or a destination to be reached. Rather, it is a state of consciousness that we can enter into at any time simply by quieting our minds and turning our attention inward.

The Role of Kriyas in Achieving Samadhi and Kundalini Awakening

Kriyas are a series of specific actions or exercises designed to cleanse the body and mind and prepare them for meditation. They are an essential part of many yoga and meditation traditions, and they can be very helpful in achieving a deeper state of consciousness. There are kriyas for every chakra, and they can be performed either individually or as a complete set. Some of the most common kriyas include pranayama (breath control), mudras (hand gestures), and bandhas (energy locks).

A. Kriyas and Samadhi

Kriyas can be very helpful in attaining a state of samadhi, as they help still the mind and focus the attention inward. They can also be used to awaken kundalini energy, which lies dormant at the base of the spine. When this energy is awakened, it rises through the chakras and brings about a state of enlightenment. Kriyas are an essential part of many yoga and meditation traditions, and they can be very helpful in achieving a deeper state of consciousness.

B. Kriyas and Kundalini Awakening

Kriyas are a common phenomenon among those who experience a Kundalini awakening. These movements may feel uncomfortable at first, but they serve a crucial purpose in the process of spiritual awakening. In general, kriyas help release tension and stagnant energy from the body and allow fresh new energy to flow more freely. They can also help keep us grounded in our physical experience while our consciousness is expanding into higher realms. Though they may be intense at times, kriyas are considered a very positive and necessary part of the Kundalini journey.

C. The Importance of Having a Teacher in Kriya Yoga

A teacher is one of the most critical aspects of any learning process, and this is especially true in the case of Kriya Yoga. In essence, Kriya Yoga is a technique for achieving spiritual enlightenment through the meditative practice of Kundalini yoga. This ancient practice has been passed down from master to student for centuries, and it requires a great deal of dedication, discipline, and guidance from an experienced teacher if it is going to be effective.

In addition to providing instruction on the various poses, breath work, and meditation techniques used in Kriya Yoga, teachers help provide emotional support and motivation. They keep students motivated when they feel discouraged or overwhelmed, helping them channel their energy into their practice while also keeping them focused on their ultimate goal - inner peace and spiritual awakening. Without these vital role models and mentors guiding us on our journey toward enlightenment, it can be easy to lose touch with ourselves and get lost along the way.

Not only do teachers and mentors play an indispensable role in passing on this ancient wisdom from generation to generation, but they also serve as guides on our journey toward self-actualization by reminding us why we started practicing in the first place. Whether you're just starting or have been practicing Kriya yoga for many years already, never underestimate the profound impact that your teacher can have on your life!

Accounts of Yogis Who Have Achieved Samadhi

There are many accounts of yogis who have achieved samadhi, or complete absorption in the divine. In this state, they report feeling a deep sense of peace, bliss, and oneness with all that is. They also often experience profound insights into the nature of reality and gain a greater understanding of the universe and our place within it.

Yoga Sutras of Patanjali

One of the most famous accounts of Samadhi comes from the Yoga Sutras of Patanjali, which is one of the most important texts on yoga and meditation. In this text, Patanjali describes eight stages of yoga, known as the ashtanga, or "eight-limbed" path. The final stage is Samadhi, which he describes as "the merging of the consciousness with the object of meditation."

Patanjali goes on to say that in this state, there is a complete cessation of the thought process and total absorption in the divine. This experience is so blissful and peaceful that it is often compared to death, as the yogi is temporarily freed from the cycle of birth and rebirth. However, unlike death, which is permanent, Samadhi is only temporary. The yogi eventually returns to a normal state of consciousness.

Swami Vivekananda

Another well-known account of samadhi comes from Swami Vivekananda, one of the most influential figures in spreading Hinduism and yoga in the West. In his autobiography, he describes an experience of

Samadhi that he had while meditating on the banks of the Ganges River.

He writes that he was "seized with a desire to know God," and he soon found himself in a state of complete absorption. In this state, he says that he lost all sense of time and space and felt an indescribable sense of peace and bliss. He also had a vision of the divine mother, whom he described as "the most beautiful thing I have ever seen."

After emerging from his meditation, Vivekananda says that he felt "a new light dawning in my soul." He also felt a deep sense of love and compassion for all beings and knew that he had been transformed by his experience.

Ramana Maharshi

One of the most famous Indian saints of the 20th century was Ramana Maharshi, who was known for his profound insights into the nature of reality. In his autobiography, he describes an experience of samadhi that happened to him when he was just a child.

He writes that he was sitting in his father's garden when he suddenly had a vision of a terrifying black snake. This vision caused him to feel intense fear, and he began to run away from the snake. However, no matter how fast he ran, the snake always seemed to be right behind him.

Finally, he came to a cliff that was too steep to climb, and he knew that the snake would catch up to him and kill him. At this moment of desperation, he had a sudden insight that there was nothing to fear, and he surrendered himself to the snake. At that moment, he says, "I lost myself. I forgot myself completely."

After this experience, Ramana Maharshi says that he felt a deep sense of peace and bliss. He also had a profound understanding of the nature of reality, and he knew that the self is not limited to the physical body.

Other Accounts

There are many other accounts of yogis who have achieved samadhi, including those of Sri Ramakrishna, Paramahansa Yogananda, and Swami Sivananda. These yogis all describe similar experiences of deep peace, bliss, and oneness with the divine. While the experiences of these yogis may seem extraordinary, anyone can achieve samadhi. With regular practice, anyone can tap into this infinite well of peace and bliss that lies within us all.

Kriya yoga is a powerful and transformative practice that has been used for thousands of years to help seekers come into direct contact with the divine. Kriya yoga aims to move beyond the ego and experience true freedom and bliss through the development of Samadhi, or deep meditative absorption. As one progresses through the stages of Kriya yoga, one may begin to awaken kundalini, an energy that is repressed by the ego and lies dormant at the base of the spine. With time, this heightened state of awareness can bring one into a more awakened state known as enlightenment or kundalini awakening. Whether you are new to Kriya yoga or have been studying it for years, this ancient practice offers countless insights, challenges, and rewards along your spiritual path.

Chapter 4: Getting Ready for the Path of Kriya

When it comes to practicing Kriya Yoga, certain prerequisites and steps must be taken to achieve success. First, you must have a good understanding of the basic tenets of yoga, such as concentration and mindfulness. Next, you must have the physical strength and flexibility to do the various poses and meditation techniques involved in this practice. Finally, you must also have the right mentality and attitude, with an open mind and an awareness of your surroundings.

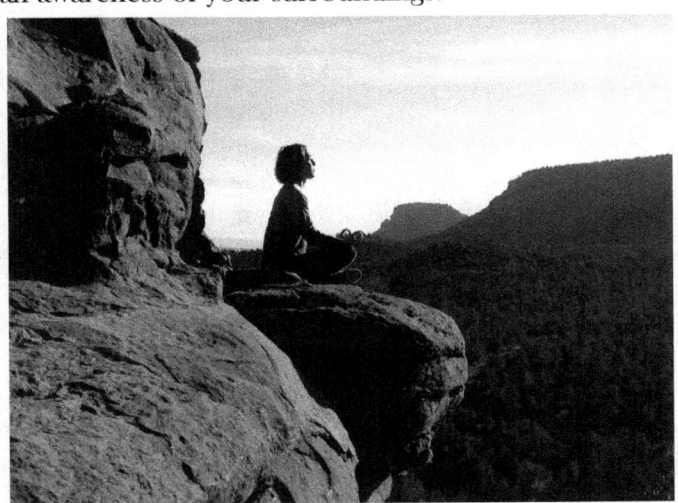

Mindfulness, concentration, and awareness are essential for preparing for Kriya.
https://pxhere.com/en/photo/1094338

For all of these reasons, doing Kriya Yoga requires some preliminary preparation before you begin your journey. With commitment and patience, you can reap many benefits from this ancient art and find greater peace within yourself. This chapter will focus on the first two limbs of yoga, the five Yamas and Niyamas. We will explore what they are, how they can help you in your Kriya Yoga practice, and how to incorporate them into your daily life.

We will also review the six Kriyas, or cleansing techniques, which are essential to this practice. Understanding and following these guidelines allows you to set yourself up for a successful and fulfilling experience with Kriya Yoga.

The Five Yamas

The Five Yamas are a set of principles that form the foundation of yoga practice, guiding yogis through their journey of self-discovery and inner peace. The first of these principles is called ahimsa, or nonviolence. This concept encourages yogis to act with compassion in every aspect of their lives, treating all human and animal beings with respect and kindness. Another Yama is asteya, or non-stealing, which calls on yogis to be mindful about how they use their time and resources. Another crucial principle is Satya, or truthfulness, which emphasizes the importance of integrity and honesty when dealing with others. These three first yamas help us cultivate kindness and compassion in ourselves and our relationships with others.

The next two yamas, however, take a slightly different approach by focusing on our relationship with ourselves rather than others. Brahmacharya is the Yama of moderation and restraint in one's actions, while aparigraha is about letting go of attachment to material things. Bringing balance into our hectic lives can be a challenge, but both brahmacharya and aparigraha can help us live more purposefully by allowing us to focus our attention on what matters most. Whether we are engaging with others or exploring our inner selves, the Five Yamas provide a road map for cultivating mindfulness and presence in all aspects of life. That makes them truly invaluable tools for anyone on the path to greater happiness and wellbeing.

1. Ahimsa - Nonviolence

Ahimsa, or nonviolence, is a central tenet of many major world religions and philosophies. This concept refers to the idea that harming others in any way, either physically or emotionally, is immoral and unethical. It can be applied on both individual and societal levels, encouraging people to practice civility and respect toward one another. There are many reasons why practicing ahimsa can be beneficial to both individuals and society as a whole. For one thing, violent behavior can often lead to negative consequences for the perpetrator as well as their victims, including physical harm, mental trauma, and social stigma. Furthermore, violence often creates greater animosity between groups of people, leading to further conflict and unrest. By choosing to practice ahimsa in all areas of life, we can help build a more peaceful society for everyone.

2. Satya - Truthfulness

Satya refers to the virtue of truthfulness and is one of the principles espoused in ancient Indian philosophy. This concept is considered especially important in yoga and meditation, as honesty and integrity are believed to be key components of spiritual evolution. Many practitioners believe that practicing Satya can help bring about lasting peace and harmony within oneself. Whether you are a yogi or just someone who values integrity, the practice of Satya can help you live your life more honestly and authentically. By striving to always stay true to yourself and your values, you can enjoy greater clarity and purpose on your path toward personal growth. If you seek peace, authenticity, and progress on your journey, then let Satya guide you.

3. Asteya - Non-Stealing

Asteya is one of the yamas, or ethical guidelines, outlined by the ancient sage Patanjali in his yoga sutras. The term asteya translates to "non-stealing," and it refers to a deep respect for other people's property. This includes physical objects and intangible things, such as ideas and time. Practicing asteya requires that we give others their due credit and refrain from taking without permission. It also encourages us to be mindful of our speech, thoughts, and actions and to ensure that they do not harm or violate others' rights. By cultivating the virtue of non-stealing, we can create a more just and harmonious world.

4. Brahmacharya - Sexual Continence

Brahmacharya, or sexual continence, is a fundamental part of many spiritual and religious traditions worldwide. This principle urges individuals to exercise restraint and discipline in their sexual practices, often refraining from sexual activity altogether or promoting celibacy as an ideal. According to proponents of this practice, abstaining from sexual activity brings a host of mental and physical benefits, including reduced stress levels, improved focus and concentration, and greater vitality and energy.

On a deeper level, the practice of brahmacharya can also be seen as an expression of one's higher self. By channeling our creative energies into noble pursuits rather than mere physical pleasures, we can more fully align ourselves with our intrinsic spiritual nature. Thus, for those who seek to grow spiritually in this way, brahmacharya represents a powerful tool for deepening that journey.

5. Aparigraha - Non-Possessiveness

At the core of yoga philosophy, yamas are intended to help guide practitioners toward a life of balance and virtue. Among these is aparigraha, or non-possessiveness, which instructs us to live simply and avoid greed and materialism. Practicing aparigraha involves letting go of what we hold dear, whether it be objects or people. We find greater peace and freedom by accepting this loss without struggle or resentment.

Furthermore, rejecting the urge to amass wealth and owning only what we need eases our overall stress level by reducing the number of possessions that need to be managed. This way, aparigraha is a powerful tool for living consciously and free from attachments. With practice, it can help yogis achieve true contentment by freeing them from their dependence on worldly things. Let go, release your hold on what you cannot always control, and embrace the power of non-possessiveness today!

The Five Niyamas

The Five Niyamas are a key component of yoga practice and form the foundation of our spiritual growth and development. Each Niyama has its distinct meaning and purpose, but they are all closely related to one another. Some scholars refer to them collectively as the "spiritual observances" given that they help us cultivate positive qualities like mindfulness, purity of thought, self-discipline, contentment, and more.

Whether you're new to yoga or have been practicing it for years, it is vital to have a deep understanding of the Five Niyamas to fully embrace their transformative power in your life. Once you've achieved that understanding, the next step is implementing this knowledge through dedicated practice and sincere efforts. When we apply ourselves diligently, we can unlock the true potential of these powerful principles and enjoy countless benefits on our journey toward growth and peace.

1. Saucha - Purity

Saucha is an essential concept in many different philosophical and spiritual traditions. At its core, *saucha* refers to the idea of purity, both physical and spiritual. Practicing saucha means maintaining a sense of clarity and calmness in one's thoughts and behavior and ensuring that one's environment is free from pollutants and distractions. Through deliberate practice, it is possible to cultivate a state of mental and emotional purity that can profoundly benefit one's overall wellbeing. Perhaps most importantly, saucha reminds us that even the smallest acts of self-care can play a vital role in our overall health and happiness. By continuously seeking out the things that bring us joy and peace of mind, we can create a truly beautiful life from the inside out.

2. Santosha - Contentment

At the heart of yogic philosophy lies the concept of *santosha* – or contentment. This state of mind is essential for living a balanced and fulfilling life, as it allows us to see things clearly without getting caught up in the distractions or illusions of modern society. When we are truly content, we are freed from the stress and worries that often accompany our daily routines, and we can appreciate all of the gifts that life has to offer. Whether we are engaged in a physical activity like yoga or simply basking in nature's beauty, practicing santosha helps us to find greater peace and happiness within ourselves. If you're looking for a way to live your best life, start cultivating an attitude of contentment today!

3. Tapasya - Austerity

Tapasya, or austerity, is a central concept in many of the major world religions. In Hinduism, for example, Tapasya is seen as a spiritual practice that allows one to come into closer contact with the divine and attain enlightenment. This may involve practicing extreme self-control and/or giving up certain worldly pleasures, such as material possessions or worldly relationships, as an act of devotion. Although different religious traditions view Tapasya differently, it is generally seen as an important and transformative part of one's spiritual journey.

Whether you are following a particular religion or simply seeking advice from a spiritual guide, guidance from someone who has undergone a significant period of self-denial can help you seek deeper meaning and find your place in the world. Suppose you're looking to cultivate greater self-discipline and explore your innermost thoughts and feelings. In that case, embarking on a journey of Tapasya may be just what you need. After all, nothing truly great comes without hard work and sacrifice!

4. Svadhyaya - Study of the Self

Svadhyaya is one of the Yamas, or moral guidelines, described in the teachings of yoga. It refers to the practice of studying and observing the self, both on a physical and spiritual level. This can encompass everything from meditating on our thoughts and feelings to practicing various breathing techniques that help us become more aware of our bodies. By constantly trying to understand ourselves better, we can learn to be more present and mindful in all aspects of our lives.

Through Svadhyaya, we can come to know ourselves on a deeper level and discover new dimensions that we may never have known existed. Whether you are just starting on your yoga journey or are an experienced practitioner, Svadhyaya is a valuable tool for growth and self-development. Whether it takes place in solitude or a group setting, this practice can help us uncover new insights about ourselves and open up a world of possibility within us.

5. Ishvara Pranidhana - Surrender to God

Ishvara Pranidhana, or surrender to God, is a key concept in many spiritual traditions. At its most basic level, Ishvara Pranidhana involves placing one's trust in a higher power and letting go of one's self-will. This can mean devoting oneself entirely to the will of God, letting go of all earthly concerns, and submitting oneself fully to divine purpose. However, this doesn't necessarily have to be an intensely religious experience. Instead, it can take on different forms depending on one's perspective.

For some, this might simply involve practicing mindfulness and meditation regularly. For others, it might involve turning inward and reconnecting with one's true self. Regardless of how one understands Ishvara Pranidhana, it is ultimately about pursuing a sense of interconnectedness with all things and recognizing that we are all part of the same larger whole.

The Six Kriyas

The ancient practice of yoga is founded on the belief that we are interconnected with all other living things and that by focusing on deepening our awareness and connection to the world around us, we can strive to become more kind, compassionate, and balanced individuals. One of the key aspects of this practice is known as the "six kriyas," or six sacred purification techniques. These practices include kapalabhati, neti, trataka, nauli, dhoti, and vasti.

Each of these methods focuses on a different part of the body and serves a unique purpose in helping us to maintain optimal health and wellbeing. For example, kapalabhati promotes healthy breathing by cleansing out the stale air from the lungs, neti washes away irritants from inside the nasal cavities, trataka helps to relieve stress by bringing attention to visual objects in our environment, nauli strengthens abdominal muscles for an improved digestive system, dhoti seeks to balance energy through slow stretching exercises, and vasti rehydrates vital organs like the kidneys and bladder.

Whether you're a seasoned yogi or new to this ancient practice, incorporating the six kriyas into your routine can help you gain deeper insight into yourself and your relationship with the wider world.

1. Kapalabhati - Skull Shining

Kapalabhati is a traditional breathing exercise from the ancient practice of yoga. It is believed to have many benefits for the body, including increased energy and improved circulation. The primary goal of Kapalabhati is to cleanse and purify the skull, and it achieves this by using forceful exhalations to expel stagnant air from the lungs. To do this technique, one simply takes a deep breath in through the nose, then exhales forcefully through the mouth while simultaneously tensing the abdomen muscles. As you continue this pattern, more and more stale air will be expelled from your lungs, allowing fresh oxygen to take its place. This can not only leave you feeling rejuvenated and refreshed, but it also helps to purify and invigorate the entire body. If you're looking for an easy way to revitalize your mind and spirit, give Kapalabhati a try today!

2. Neti - Nasal Cleansing

Neti is a popular method of nasal cleansing that has been used for centuries in many different cultures. This technique involves pouring water or saline solution into one nostril and letting it flow out through the other, clearing away dust, pollen, and other irritants. One major benefit of neti is that it can help to relieve congestion and improve airflow through the sinuses, helping to relieve allergies and other respiratory conditions. In addition, some research has shown that regular use of neti may help to boost your immune system, protecting you from unwanted bacteria and viruses. Overall, whether you are looking for relief from allergies or just want to stay healthy year-round, neti is an excellent tool for keeping your sinuses clear and healthy. With simple instructions that anyone can follow at home, it's never been easier to reap all the benefits of this traditional remedy.

To practice neti, you'll need a neti pot or another similar device. Fill the pot with lukewarm water or saline solution, and then tilt your head to the side so that one nostril is pointing down towards the pot. Slowly pour the water or solution into this nostril, and allow it to flow out through the other nostril. You may need to breathe through your mouth during this process. Repeat on the other side, and then rinse out your mouth and nose with clean water when finished.

3. Trataka - Candle Gazing

Trataka, or candle gazing, is a form of meditation that has been practiced for centuries in many different cultures. This simple practice involves staring at a flame or other object to clear the mind and focus your attention on the present moment. To begin, you simply sit comfortably in a quiet place and gaze at the light of a candle, focusing all of your attention on the flickering flame. As you do this, you may notice that thoughts and sensations from the outside world gradually fade from your awareness. You are left with just the light – pure and simple – filling your entire consciousness. Over time, practicing trataka can help you better cultivate presence and mindfulness in your daily life, making you more aware of each moment as it passes.

4. Nauli - Abdominal Massage

Nauli is a type of abdominal massage that has been practiced in India for hundreds of years. This unique form of massage involves massaging and twisting the abdominal muscles to loosen them, promoting better circulation and improved digestive function. According to ancient texts, nauli was used by yogis and spiritual practitioners as a way to cleanse their internal organs and increase energy levels. This practice continues to be used for physical and spiritual benefits. To perform nauli, begin by standing with your feet hip-width apart. Place your hands on your lower belly, and take a deep breath in. As you exhale, contract your abdominal muscles to the best of your ability. Then, using your hands as a guide, move these contracted muscles from side to side in a massaging motion. Finally, twist the muscles in a clockwise and counterclockwise direction. Repeat this process for several minutes, and then release the contraction and take a few deep breaths.

5. Dhoti - Intestinal Wash

The dhoti, or intestinal wash, is one of the most popular traditional remedies for treating many health conditions. In addition to soothing problems like cramping and upset stomach, regular use of the dhoti can also help improve overall digestion and boost overall immune function. This practice involves swallowing a piece of cloth soaked in warm water or herbal tea. Once the cloth is inside the stomach, it has to remain there for a short time before being removed. Many people practicing the dhoti say it is an incredibly effective way to cleanse the digestive system and promote gut health. However, for beginners, it is crucial to have an instructor or an experienced practitioner present during the process for safety purposes. Consult your doctor before trying this.

6. Vasti - Bladder Wash

Vasti is a common treatment for a variety of bladder diseases and disorders. This ancient practice involves washing the bladder with water to clean out any impurities that may be present. While it may not sound like the most pleasant experience, it can greatly benefit your health and wellbeing. It involves standing waist-deep in water and allowing the water to enter through the urethra and fill the bladder. Once the bladder is full, the water is then released through the urethra. This process is repeated several times until the water is clear. Vasti reduces inflammation and pain associated with bladder conditions while also helping to increase circulation in the area. Furthermore, this treatment can help to balance the body's natural pH levels, restoring the proper functioning of all your bodily systems.

When it comes to getting ready for the path of kriya, it is essential to first understand the basics of the five yamas and niyamas. These are the foundation of yoga and provide the framework for a healthy and harmonious life. This chapter has provided you with an overview of these crucial concepts and tips on how to incorporate them into your daily life. Before moving on to the next section, take some time to reflect on how you can incorporate the yamas and niyamas into your own life. What changes can you make to your daily routine to align with these principles? How can you bring more awareness to your thoughts and actions? Remember, the goal is not to perfect these concepts but rather to use them as a guide on your journey to self-discovery.

Chapter 5: Pranayama: The Art of Breathing

Breathing is an essential function of life, but it's also something we often take for granted. We breathe automatically and don't give it much thought - that is, until we start experiencing shortness of breath. When that happens, it's a reminder of just how important our respiratory system is. The ancient practice of Yoga includes a variety of breath control exercises known as pranayama. These exercises can improve lung function and increase overall vitality. They can also be used as a tool for managing stress and anxiety.

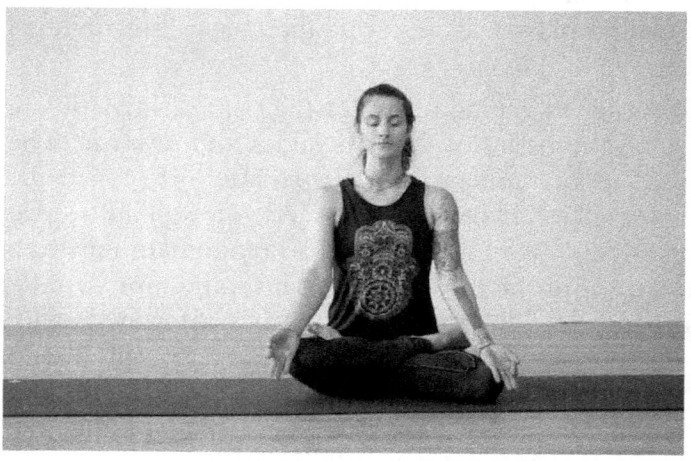

Mastering the art of breathing is essential to reach a state of inner peace.
https://unsplash.com/photos/9aoIPynE26U

What Is Pranayama?

Pranayama is a branch of Yoga that focuses on breath control. The goal of pranayama is to help practitioners achieve a state of calm and inner peace. The word pranayama is derived from two Sanskrit words, "prana," which means life force or energy, and "ayama," which means control or regulation. Many different techniques can be used to practice pranayama. One popular method is Alternate Nostril Breathing, which involves inhaling and exhaling through each nostril in turn. This type of breathing is said to help balance the left and right hemispheres of the brain, promoting a sense of calm and clarity. Other benefits of pranayama include improved respiratory function, reduced stress and anxiety, and increased focus and concentration. Remember, the key to reaping the benefits of pranayama is regular practice. Like any skill, it takes time and effort to master. With patience and perseverance, you'll be on your way to achieving inner peace in no time.

The pranayama cycle has three phases, puraka (inhalation), kumbhaka (retention), and rechaka (exhalation). Each phase plays an important role in the overall practice of pranayama, and each one can be further divided into sub-phases.

- Puraka, or inhalation, is the first phase of the pranayama cycle. The purpose of puraka is to fill the lungs with fresh air, providing the body with oxygen and energy. During puraka, the breath is slowly and deliberately inhaled through the nose, filling the lungs from bottom to top. Once the lungs are full, the breath is held briefly before moving on to kumbhaka.
- Kumbhaka, or retention, is the second phase of pranayama. During kumbhaka, the breath is held in the lungs, allowing the body to absorb more oxygen. Kumbhaka can be further divided into two sub-phases: antara kumbhaka, done with the glottis closed, and bahya kumbhaka, done with the glottis open. Both types of kumbhaka are important for different reasons. Antara kumbhaka helps to build internal heat, while bahya kumbhaka cools and refreshes the body.
- Rechaka, or exhalation, is the third and final phase of pranayama. The purpose of rechaka is to expel all of the air from the lungs so that they can be filled with fresh air during Puraka. Rechaka should be done slowly and deliberately through the nose,

emptying the lungs from top to bottom. Once all of the air has been exhaled, Puraka can begin again.

What Is Prana Breathing?

Breathing is an important part of our daily lives. We need it to live, yet we often take it for granted. However, there are many different ways to breathe, and each has its own benefits. One way to improve your breathing is to practice prana breathing, also known as abdominal breathing or belly breathing. This type of breathing increases the flow of prana, or life force energy, throughout the body. This type of breathing encourages full oxygen exchange by expanding the diaphragm and lungs. It also massages the internal organs and helps release body tension. It improves mental clarity and focus and boosts physical energy levels. Prana breathing is also thought to help detoxify the body and promote a sense of calm and wellbeing.

To practice prana breathing, sit with your spine straight and place one hand on your belly. Breathe in slowly through your nose, allowing your belly to expand. Breathe out fully through your mouth. Repeat this for a few minutes, letting your body relax deeper with each inhale and exhale. You may want to close your eyes and focus on the sensation of your breath moving in and out of your body. When you're finished, sit for a few moments and notice how you feel. Most people find that prana breathing is calming and invigorating, and it can be done anywhere, anytime. Give it a try next time you're feeling stressed or in need of a quick energy boost.

Why Is Mastering Pranayama Important?

Kriya Yoga and meditation are two spiritual practices that are said to lead to enlightenment. In order to achieve the highest level of spiritual development, it is said that one must master pranayam, which is the control of breath. Pranayam is said to be the key to unlocking the door to higher states of consciousness. When performed correctly, it is said to help purify the mind and body and promote physical and mental health. There are many different types of pranayam, each with its own benefits. For example, kapalbhati pranayam (breath of fire) cleanses the respiratory system, while bhastrika pranayam (bellows breath) improves circulation and increases energy levels. Mastering pranayam takes time and practice, but those who do so are said to reap great rewards.

What Are the Health Benefits of Pranayama?

1. Cognitive Function

Yoga and meditation have been shown to be beneficial for overall health, but did you know that specific breathing exercises, known as pranayama, can also improve cognitive function? Pranayama can improve memory, attention span, and reaction time. In addition, pranayama reduces stress levels and improves emotional wellbeing. While the exact mechanism is not fully understood just yet, it is believed that pranayama works by increasing the supply of oxygen to the brain. If you're looking for a way to boost your brain power, give pranayama a try.

2. Lung Capacity

There are many different types of pranayama, but all involve breath control in some way. Practitioners believe that pranayama can have numerous benefits, including increased lung capacity and improved circulation. Additionally, pranayama is said to be beneficial for people with asthma and other respiratory disorders. While no scientific evidence supports these claims, many people continue to practice pranayama regularly to improve their overall health and wellbeing.

3. Quitting Smoking

Pranayam has many benefits, including improving lung function and increasing oxygen intake. Additionally, it has been shown to help people quit smoking and recover from smoking-related damage. It helps with cleansing the lungs and improving lung function. It also increases oxygen intake and improves circulation. Additionally, pranayam reduces stress and anxiety, both of which are common triggers for smoking. Finally, pranayam can help repair damaged cells and tissues in the lungs, making it an effective tool for recovering from smoking-related damage.

4. Mindfulness

Pranayam is said to be especially beneficial for mindfulness. It consists of a series of breathing exercises that help control breathing. This, in turn, is said to help control the mind. In our fast-paced, modern world, it can be easy to get caught up in our thoughts and forget to pay attention to the present moment. By focusing on our breath, we can learn to focus our attention on the present and let go of distractions. This can lead to a more mindful and peaceful state of mind. Therefore, it may be worth incorporating some pranayam into your daily routine if you are looking for ways to improve your mindfulness and overall health.

5. Stress and Emotional Regulation

Pranayam is an ancient practice used for centuries to help promote physical and mental wellbeing. While it has many benefits, one of the most well-known is its ability to help regulate stress and emotions. When we are under stress, our bodies produce hormones that can negatively affect our health. Over time, chronic stress can lead to serious health problems such as anxiety, depression, heart disease, and more. By practicing pranayam regularly, we can keep our stress levels in check and prevent negative health effects.

Additionally, pranayam has been shown to help manage emotions such as anger and frustration. By learning how to control our breath, we can better control our emotions and react more positively to stressful situations. Overall, the benefits of pranayam are numerous and can profoundly affect your health and wellbeing.

6. Psychosomatic disorders

Pranayam is an ancient breathing technique practiced for centuries in India. There are many benefits of pranayam, including reducing stress, improving circulation, and helping to tackle psychosomatic disorders. Additionally, pranayam is effective in treating psychosomatic disorders such as migraine headaches, ulcers, and psoriasis

Types of Pranayama

There are many different types of pranayama, but they can broadly be divided into two categories: purifying and energizing breaths. Purifying breaths are designed to cleanse the body and remove toxins. They typically involve exhaling for longer than you inhale. Energizing breaths are designed to increase energy levels and promote alertness. They typically involve inhaling for longer than you exhale. Both types of pranayama can be beneficial, but it's important to start slowly and build up gradually. If you're new to pranayama, it's best to practice under the guidance of an experienced teacher. Once you've mastered the basics, you can practice at home whenever you need a little boost of energy or calmness.

Kriya Pranayama Techniques

Kapal Bhati Pranayama

Kapalbhati pranayama is a type of breathing exercise that originates from Yoga. It is also known as Skull Shining Breath or Breathing Through the Forehead. The name comes from the Sanskrit words "kapala," meaning skull, and "bhati," meaning light. Thus, the practice's name literally means "skull shining breath." It is often used as a preparatory exercise for other Yoga practices, such as meditation and pranayama. This pranayama is said to cleanse the lungs and sinuses, improve concentration and memory, and reduce stress and anxiety. It is also said to benefit the liver, kidneys, and digestive system.

Steps:
1. Sit in a comfortable position with your spine straight.
2. Place your hands on your knees with your palms facing up. Close your eyes and take a deep breath through your nose.
3. The belly is then sucked in, so the navel moves toward the spine.
4. A deep inhalation is taken, and then the exhale is initiated by pushing all of the air out through the nose while drawing the navel back towards the spine.
5. As you exhale, forcefully contract your abdominal muscles and exhale through your nose with a hissing sound.
6. Continue this rapid breathing for 10-15 minutes. Then, slowly exhale and relax your body.

You can practice this pranayama once or twice a day.

Kapal Bhati pranayama is said to have many benefits, including improved respiratory function, increased energy levels, reduced stress levels, and improved digestion. Some people also believe that it can help improve mental clarity and focus. Improper technique can lead to dizziness, nausea, or hyperventilation.

Kapal and Karna Randhra Dhauti

Kapal randhra dhauti kriya is a yogic cleansing technique used to cleanse the sinuses and improve brain function. The name comes from the Sanskrit words kapala, meaning "skull," and randhra, meaning "hole." Dhauti means "to cleanse." To do this kriya, sit comfortably with your eyes closed. Kapal randhra dhauti kriya is a simple but effective technique that can be done daily to cleanse the sinuses and improve brain function.

This practice is said to help treat conditions such as allergies, colds, sinus infections, and headaches.

Steps:
1. Sit in a comfortable position with your spine straight.
2. Rest your elbows on your knees and close your eyes.
3. Using your thumb and forefinger, gently massage the inner corners of your eyes.
4. Gently press your temples with your thumbs and index fingers while lightly touching your skull with your other fingers.
5. Then, press firmly on the space between your eyebrows using your middle finger.
6. Finally, cup your hands over your mouth and nose and inhale deeply through your nose. Exhale slowly through your mouth. Repeat this process for several minutes.

Kapal and Karna Randhra Dhauti can be performed once or twice a day for the best results.

Dog Breathing

Dog Breathing Kriya is a breathing exercise that is said to be beneficial for both physical and mental health. The basic premise of the kriya is that by breathing deeply and slowly, one can help to improve the function of the internal organs and calm the mind. There are a number of different ways to perform Dog Breathing Kriya, but all involve inhaling and exhaling in a slow and controlled manner. Some people may find it helpful to practice the kriya for several minutes each day, while others may only need to do it on occasion. Regardless of how often it is done, Dog Breathing Kriya offers various benefits, including improved circulation, reduced stress levels, and enhanced mental clarity. When performed correctly, it can improve lung capacity and respiratory function, as well as reducing stress and promoting relaxation. Here's how to do it:

Steps:
1. Sit in a comfortable position with your spine straight and your eyes closed.
2. Place your hands on your thighs, palms down.
3. Take a deep breath through your nose, then exhale forcefully through your mouth. Make an "ahh" sound as you exhale.

4. Continue breathing this way for several rounds, then return to normal breathing.
5. To finish, take a few deep breaths and feel the energy of the kriya circulating through your body.

PET- Pranic Energization Technique

PET, or Pranic Energization Technique, is a simple but effective healing method that anyone can learn. It involves using the hands to draw universal life force energy, or prana, to the body. This can be done for oneself or others and is said to be helpful for many physical and emotional ailments. PET is based on the belief that a build-up of negative energy in the body causes all illness. By clearing this energy and infusing the body with fresh prana, PET can promote healing. The technique is said to be particularly beneficial for conditions that are chronic or difficult to treat. While PET is not a cure-all, it can be a helpful addition to any healing toolkit.

PET, or the Pranic Energization Technique, is a simple yet effective way to cleanse and energize the body. It involves using the hands to lightly massage the head and draw energy from the environment. The process is said to clear away negative energy and promote healing. Here is a step-by-step guide to performing PET:

Steps:
1. Start by standing in a comfortable position with your feet shoulder-width apart. Place your palms on your lower abdomen, just below the navel.
2. Draw in a deep breath and exhale slowly, allowing your stomach to expand as you breathe out.
3. As you inhale again, visualize a ball of white light forming in your hands.
4. Once the ball of light is bright and strong, begin massaging your head with your palms, using gentle circular motions. Start at the forehead and move down to the temples and back of the neck. Spend extra time on any areas that feel tense or bloated.
5. Continue massaging for about two minutes, then slowly release the ball of light back into the environment. Repeat as needed.

Rabbit Breathing

For centuries, meditation has been used to promote mental and physical wellbeing. If you're feeling stressed, you might want to try the

Rabbit Breathing Exercise. This type of meditation is based on the teachings of the Buddhist monk Thich Nhat Hanh, and it can help you to focus and calm your mind. In recent years, this technique gained popularity for its ability to promote relaxation and ease anxiety. Rabbit breathing is simple but effective and can be done anywhere at any time.

Steps:
1. Simply sit in a comfortable position and close your eyes.
2. Then, take a deep breath in through your nose and out through your mouth.
3. As you exhale, imagine that your stomach is a balloon filled with air.
4. Continue to breathe deeply and slowly, allowing your stomach to expand with each breath.
5. As you exhale, imagine all of your stress and tension leaving your body.
6. Continue this deep breathing for several minutes or until you feel calm and relaxed.

Rabbit breathing is an excellent way to reduce stress and anxiety, and it can also be used as a tool to help you fall asleep at night. Give it a try the next time you need a break from the hustle and bustle of life.

Bhastrika Pranayama

Bhastrika pranayama is a Yoga breathing exercise that involves forcefully exhaling and inhaling through the nose. The name comes from the Sanskrit words bhasta, meaning "bellows," and ika, meaning "small." Bhastrika pranayama is also sometimes called "bellows breath." Bhastrika pranayama is said to clear the sinuses, improve lung function, and increase energy levels. It is also thought to help relieve anxiety and stress. Bhastrika pranayama is generally considered safe for healthy people. However, it may not be suitable for people with high blood pressure or heart conditions.

Steps:
1. Sit in a comfortable position with your spine straight. Place your hands on your knees with your palms facing down.
2. Close your eyes and take a few deep breaths.
3. Then, begin exhaling and inhaling forcefully through your nose.
4. Continue for 30 seconds to 1 minute.

5. You can then return to normal breathing and open your eyes.

Nadi Shodhana Pranayama

Nadis are energy channels in the body through which Prana, or life force energy, flows. Shodhana means purification. Therefore, Nadi Shodhana Pranayama is a breathing exercise that purifies the body's energy channels. There are three main nadis, or energy channels, in the body, ida, pingala, and sushumna. Ida and pingala run along either side of the spine and correspond to the left and right nostrils. Sushumna runs along the center of the spine and is associated with the third eye or Ajna chakra. Nadi Shodhana Pranayama alternates breathing between the left and right nostrils to purify and balance the body's energy flow.

Steps:
1. Sit in a comfortable position with your spine straight.
2. Rest your left hand on your left knee in Jnana Mudra (index finger and thumb touching) with your right hand in Vishnu Mudra (right thumb resting on top of left index finger).
3. Close your right nostril with your right thumb and inhale deeply through your left nostril.
4. Then close your left nostril with your ring finger and exhale slowly through your right nostril.
5. Inhale again through your right nostril and then close it off with your thumb.
6. Exhale through your left nostril.
7. This completes one cycle of Nadi Shodhana Pranayama. Continue for 5-10 minutes, alternating breathing between the left and right nostrils.

Now that you know everything about pranayama and how it can complement kriya, it's time to start practicing! Master this breathing technique, and you'll soon see the benefits for yourself. With regular practice, you will notice an improvement in your energy levels, concentration, and overall wellbeing.

Chapter 6: Mudras and Mantras

Kriya Yoga is a system of meditation that uses various mudras, hand gestures, and mantras to help practitioners deepen their practice. Mudras are an essential part of Kriya Yoga because they help channel energy flow in the body and can target specific areas for healing. In addition, mantras are often recited to help focus the mind and connect with the divine. This chapter will explore the benefits of mudras and mantras and provide instructions for some of the most common mudras and mantras used in Kriya Yoga.

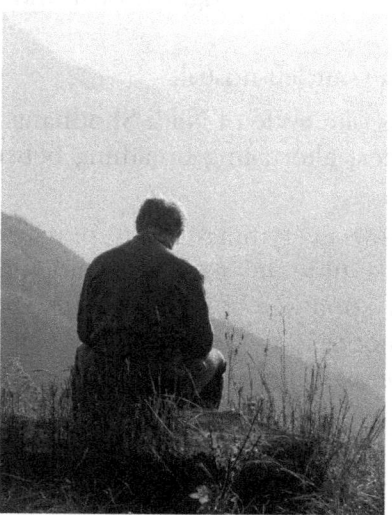

Using gestures and recitation stimulates the brain for meditation.
Photo by Lisa van Vliet on Unsplash https://unsplash.com/photos/a-man-sitting-on-top-of-a-hill-overlooking-a-valley-E04T3VI8KoI

Mudras

Mudras are a type of hand gesture used in many different types of spiritual and religious practices. These gestures are believed to have special powers. They stimulate particular areas of the brain and facilitate various mental and physical processes. In many cases, mudras are used in conjunction with meditation or breathing exercises to create a sense of balance and wellbeing. Depending on the specific practice, mudras may be done with the hands facing up, down, or in other positions. Along with practicing mudras individually, they can also be incorporated into other activities, such as Yoga or dance. Overall, mudras offer a unique and powerful way to connect with one's inner self and achieve greater levels of health and wellbeing.

Benefits of Mudras

Mudras are a unique and powerful practice that can have many benefits for the body, mind, and spirit. These simple hand gestures work by activating specific points in the body, which can help stimulate healing processes and improve overall health. Additionally, mudras help to cultivate mindfulness and reduce stress, encouraging greater mental clarity and peace of mind. Whether used as part of meditation or simply performed throughout the day as needed, mudras offer a valuable tool for cultivating wellbeing at all levels. Here are some of the most common benefits associated with practicing mudras:

A. Improved Circulation

Controlling the flow of energy through the body is essential for good health. Many people experience problems with circulation, which can result in pain, fatigue, and even restricted blood flow to the heart and brain. One effective way to improve circulation is through mudras, which can help to stimulate certain areas of the body. These ancient techniques use a combination of pressure, movement, and focus on stimulating different energy pathways throughout the body. This encourages healthy circulation by opening up blocked channels and clearing out stagnant energy. In addition, mudras are easy to incorporate into daily life, making them a practical and effective way to promote better circulation and overall wellbeing.

B. Increased Serotonin Levels

Mudras are simple hand gestures that can be used to engage certain energy centers in the body. By focusing on certain patterns of finger positioning and using these as a kind of physical meditation practice, we can increase our levels of serotonin, a chemical responsible for regulating mood and feelings of calmness and happiness. Because mudras work in such a direct way to affect our mental state, they are a highly effective tool for managing stress, anxiety, and depression. When you're feeling overwhelmed at work or dealing with the usual frustrations of daily life, a few minutes spent practicing your favorite mudra can help to uplift your spirit and restore your sense of peace and balance.

C. Relief from Pain

As anyone who deals with chronic pain knows, it can be a very challenging and debilitating condition. If you have had to deal with this kind of pain for a long time, you may have tried various medications or therapies in search of relief. One alternative treatment you may not have heard of is the practice of mudras. In simple terms, mudras are physical gestures that are believed to have a therapeutic effect on the body and mind. These hand positions are thought to stimulate certain points on the body and activate the flow of energy within the body, which may help reduce pain and tension. While more research is needed to confirm the full efficacy of these hand positions, there is some evidence that they can be an effective tool for dealing with pain.

D. Improved Digestion

Mudras are simple hand gestures that have been used for centuries in Yoga and meditation practices. Often used to focus the mind or invoke specific energies, mudras can offer a range of health benefits to the body and mind. Perhaps one of the most overlooked benefits of these fascinating gestures is their ability to improve digestion. By activating certain pressure points in the hands, mudras can stimulate certain organs and promote better circulation, resulting in improved digestive function. Whether you're an experienced yogi or just looking for a natural way to boost your overall wellbeing, incorporating mudras into your routine can help you achieve better digestive health and enjoy all the benefits that come with it.

E. Better Sleep

Sleep is essential to good health, allowing our bodies and minds to rest and recharge after a long day. For many people, getting a good night's sleep can be challenging. Luckily, mudras have several physical benefits, including boosting brain function and enhancing relaxation. Perhaps one of the most well-known mudras is called the "Gyan mudra." This mudra involves holding the tip of your thumb to the tip of your index finger while keeping your other fingers straight and parallel to each other. Many people practice this mudra before going to bed to promote better sleep, as it has a calming effect on both body and mind. If you're having trouble sleeping at night, try incorporating some mudras into your evening routine!

Meaning, Benefits, and Instructions for Common Mudras

Though they may seem like simple movements, mudras can offer a range of physical and mental benefits. Here are some of the most common mudras and their benefits:

A. Buddha Mudra

Buddha mudra, also known as the gesture of meditation or bestowing gifts, is widely recognized as one of the most important and meaningful hand gestures in Yoga and Buddhist practices. According to tradition, this powerful mudra can be used to boost mental clarity and focus, reduce stress and anxiety, and promote feelings of calmness and wellbeing. It can also help remove obstacles from our path and stimulate positive energy wherever it is directed.

To begin practicing Buddha mudra, start by sitting comfortably in a cross-legged position with your hands resting gently on your thighs. Next, place the tips of your index fingers together so that they resemble a stylized lotus bud, a metaphor for enlightenment. Then, extend your middle fingers out so that they are pointing straight up toward the sky. Finally, hold your other fingers loosely curled against the palm of each hand.

While many different variations of Buddha mudra are available, this hand gesture should always be performed with proper alignment and mindfulness to achieve its full benefits. Take time to visualize what you hope to gain from engaging in Buddha mudra and let go of any negative thoughts that arise during this process. With regular practice, you'll find greater satisfaction and peace in your daily life and discover new sources of inspiration when dealing with adversity or uncertainty.

B. Gyan Mudra

Gyan Mudra is a Yoga posture used for both physical and mental benefits. Its name comes from the Sanskrit words for "awareness" and "thumb," referring to the contact between the thumb and index or middle finger. Practicing this posture has been shown to improve focus, regulate breathing, and improve circulation, as well as provide some protection against disease. To perform this pose, gently press your thumb against the tip of either your index or middle finger and hold it there for five to ten minutes, then repeat with the other arm. If you are new to Yoga, start by practicing Gyan Mudra in short intervals at first before gradually increasing the duration over time. With consistent practice, this posture can help you achieve better health and enhanced awareness of both yourself and your surroundings.

C. Surya Mudra

Surya Mudra, also known as the Mudra of the Sun, is an ancient hand gesture that has been practiced for centuries in both Indian and Chinese yogic traditions. This mudra involves bringing the ring finger and thumb of one hand into a ring shape as if forming a fist while extending the other three fingers out straight. The benefits of this gesture are numerous, ranging from improved digestion and lower stress levels to increased physical energy, better mental clarity, and even enhanced immunity.

To perform Surya Mudra, begin by sitting comfortably with your spine erect and then bring the ring finger and thumb of your right hand together in front of your chest while keeping the other three fingers extended straight. Next, tilt your head slightly to the right while focusing on your nose or third eye area. Hold this position for 5-10 minutes, breathing deeply and consciously throughout. As you practice Surya Mudra regularly, you will notice more sustained energy levels and a greater sense of mental calmness and clarity. Best of all, this graceful gesture can be practiced anywhere at any time for maximum results!

D. Prana Mudra

Prana mudra, also known as the energy gesture, is one of many different types of tantric hand gestures that can be used to manipulate energy or prana within the body. Prana mudra is typically performed by joining the tips of the ring and index fingers together while keeping the other three fingers straight and relaxed. This mudra is held with both hands, typically along with a few other modifications of hand positions. The benefits of prana mudra depend on its specific application, but it is generally thought to have a calming and energizing effect. It also helps in overcoming stress and anxiety, promoting circulation and healing, and enhancing focus and concentration.

To perform prana mudra, start by sitting in a comfortable position with your shoulders down and relaxed. Extend your arms out parallel to your torso, palms facing downward. Next, fold your middle two fingers inward so that the tips touch each other tightly. Finally, connect the tip of your thumb with the tip of either your middle or ring finger. Hold this pose for 2-3 minutes at a time as you breathe deeply in and out through your nose.

E. Shankh Mudra

The shankh mudra is one of the most effective ways to boost your energy, increase mental clarity, and improve circulation throughout the body. This simple hand position draws energy into the hands, allowing you to take in the benefits of prana, or life force energy. In addition, practicing this mudra can help to calm the mind and alleviate stress, making it an ideal way to begin or end a meditation session.

To perform the shankh mudra, simply place your palms together so that your thumbs are directly touching each other. Make sure that all fingers are pointing straight up, with your thumb on top of your index finger from both hands. Hold this position for at least 30 seconds to start feeling the benefits of this powerful mudra. With regular practice, you can gain even more benefits from this simple yet powerful hand gesture. You'll be amazed by how energized and focused you feel after just a few minutes.

F. Hakini Mudra

Hakini Mudra, also known as the Seal of Wisdom, is a practice that yogis around the world have used for thousands of years. This powerful mudra involves bringing your hands together and bringing your thumb, index finger, and middle finger in contact with each other. This mudra is said to bring clarity and wisdom, opening up channels of spiritual energy throughout your body. In addition, Hakini Mudra can help build focus and concentration by facilitating the flow of oxygen and blood throughout your brain. To do this mudra properly, you should hold it for several minutes at a time without any distractions or breaks. Some people find that this pose enhances meditation and improves overall wellbeing.

G. Kamal Mudra

Kamal Mudra is a powerful hand gesture that is said to offer a range of mental and physical benefits. Also known as Lotus Seal, this mudra involves making a fist with the left hand and then extending the fingers to touch the tip of the thumb. This forms a lotus flower shape with the fingertips, which has been associated with wisdom and clarity of mind in various cultures and traditions. By practicing Kamal Mudra regularly, you can enhance your ability to focus and increase your stress resilience, helping you feel more relaxed and at ease in any situation.

Additionally, because this mudra stimulates certain nerves along the palm, it can also have an impact on pain levels and overall energy levels. To get started, simply sit comfortably with your hands resting on your lap. Curl your left hand into a loose fist. Extend your fingers, so they touch the tip of your thumb. Hold this position for up to five minutes at a time while focusing on slow, deep breathing. Repeat as often as you like each day. With regular practice, you'll immediately start seeing the benefits of Kamal Mudra!

Mantras

Mantras are special phrases or words we use to help focus our minds and bring inner peace. Often associated with spirituality and religion, mantras can be found in many different traditions and belief systems. Whether it's a word repeated silently in your head or a phrase spoken out loud, a mantra can be used at any time of day to positively influence your thoughts and emotions. Whether you're seeking more serenity in your life or simply looking for an effective way to ground yourself amid the chaos of modern life, using mantras is an excellent tool for finding peace within yourself.

A. So Ham

The So Ham mantra is a simple yet effective meditation tool that has been used for centuries to help practitioners deepen their self-awareness, improve focus, and increase mental clarity. Also known as the Sound of Silence or the Secret Name of God, the mantra consists of just three simple syllables, so, ham, and om. Each syllable represents a different aspect of our being – our bodies (so), our minds (ham), and our spirit (om). By repeating this mantra in meditation, we can reconnect with all parts of ourselves, ultimately creating more balance and harmony in our inner lives and external experiences.

B. Hare Krishna

The Hare Krishna mantra, also known as the Maha-Mantra, is a potent meditation tool that has been practiced for centuries in Hinduism and other spiritual traditions. This sacred mantra invokes the divine energy of the Supreme Lord, or Krishna, as well as his most devoted devotee, Radha. The chanting of this mantra is believed to have many physical and spiritual benefits, including equanimity of mind, improved concentration and memory, protection from negative energies and forces, and more. Whether you are looking to deepen your spiritual practice or embark on a new journey of self-exploration, there is no better way to connect with the divine than through learning and practicing the beckoning call of this beloved chant: *"Hare Krishna Hare Krishna; Krishna Krishna Hare Hare; Hare Rama Hare Rama; Rama Rama Hare Hare!"*

C. Om Namah Shivaya

The Om Namah Shivaya mantra is one of the most well-known and widely used Hindu mantras. This sacred chant is dedicated to the Hindu god Shiva and serves as a powerful way to reconnect with this deity. To fully understand the meaning and benefits of Om Namah Shivaya, consider its translation. In Sanskrit, the mantra translates to *"I bow down to the Infinite One."* Through this simple phrase, we are recognizing the universe's limitless, all-encompassing nature, acknowledging all its aspects as part of our being.

Beyond its spiritual significance, many physical benefits are associated with reciting this ancient mantra. Studies have shown that Om Namah Shivaya can help lower heart rate and blood pressure, relieve anxiety, and improve sleep quality. As a result, many people use this chant as a tool for relaxation or stress management. Whether you use it as a spiritual practice or a means of promoting health and wellness, Om Namah Shivaya is sure to provide deep healing and transformative benefits for anyone who embraces it with an open heart and mind.

D. Gayatri Mantra

The Gayatri Mantra is one of the most widely-recited prayers in Hinduism and other Indian religions. This ancient mantra holds a special significance for many people, as it is believed to have transformative power and bring blessings upon those who recite it. The mantra has a poetic, beautiful quality, with each line seeking to invoke different aspects of the divine. However, for those unfamiliar with the meaning of this sacred text, understanding its translation and meaning can help unlock its full potential. Here is a translation of the Gayatri Mantra:

"Om bhur bhuvah svah; tat savitur varennyam; bhargo devasya dhimahi; dhiyo yo nah prachodayat"

This mantra can be translated to mean: *"We meditate on the divine light of the creator; may that enlighten our minds."* Through this simple prayer, we are asking for guidance and wisdom from the divine source.

The Gayatri Mantra is traditionally recited 21 times a day, and there are many benefits associated with this practice. Some of these benefits include increased concentration and mental clarity, improved self-esteem and confidence, and a deeper connection to the divine. Through chanting its powerful words, we can channel divine energy and gain insight into our truths.

Reciting this mantra can also help us make important choices in life, giving us the courage and strength we need to follow our heart's true path. In addition, incorporating the practice of this mantra into our daily routines can strengthen our focus and discipline by helping us enter a deep state of meditation that transcends all worldly distractions. Overall, whether you are looking for guidance in your spiritual journey or simply want to experience the profound beauty of one of Hinduism's greatest esoteric texts, there is likely something valuable you can glean from reciting the Gayatri Mantra.

E. Maha Mrityunjaya Mantra

The Maha Mrityunjaya Mantra, or "Great Death-Defeating Mantra," is one of the most powerful mantras in Hinduism. It is said to offer protection from death and disease, and it has been used for thousands of years by yogis and spiritual practitioners to promote healing and longevity. The exact meaning of the mantra is somewhat ambiguous, but it is generally believed to refer to Lord Shiva as the destroyer who can bring about both death and new life. Here is a translation of the Maha Mrityunjaya Mantra:

"Om tryambakam yajamahe sugandhim pushtivardhanam; urvarukam iva bandhanan mrityor mukshiya mamritat"

This mantra can be translated to mean: *"We worship the three-eyed Lord who is fragrant and who nourishes all beings. May He free us from death for the sake of immortality, just as the cucumber is freed from its bondage when it is separated from the vine."*

This mantra calls upon the ancient Vedic gods Indra and Agni to act as protectors against all forms of harm. Through repeated chanting and meditation on these themes, practitioners are believed to receive tremendous benefits that help them live long, healthy lives. Whether chanted alone or in a group setting, the Maha Mrityunjaya Mantra is a powerful tool for promoting wellness, both physical and spiritual.

Mantras and mudras are both important aspects of Kriya Yoga and meditation. Each has its unique benefits that can help practitioners to improve their practice. By incorporating these techniques into your daily routine, you can experience improved concentration, mental clarity, and a deeper connection to the divine. The mantras and mudras featured in this chapter are just a few of the many that are available. As you explore these practices further, allow yourself to be open to new experiences and discover which ones work best for you.

Chapter 7: Kriya Meditation Techniques

Kriya Yoga is an ancient system of meditation first expounded by the sage Patanjali in the Yoga Sutras. The word "Kriya" literally means "action" or "activities," and it refers to a set of techniques designed to promote inner stillness and spiritual awakening. Kriya Yoga is often referred to as the "Yoga of awareness," as it helps practitioners become more aware of their thoughts, feelings, and actions.

There are many different Kriya meditation techniques, but some of the most common include pranayama (breath control), mantra recitation, and visualization. Kriya Yoga can be practiced alone or in groups, and there are many different schools that offer instruction in this type of meditation. However, it is important to remember that Kriya Yoga is not a religion, and anyone can learn and practice these techniques regardless of their beliefs.

How Important Is Meditation in Kriya Yoga?

1. Assists in Self Realization

Meditation is an important part of Kriya Yoga because it helps practitioners realize their true nature. When we meditate, we turn our attention inward and focus on our breath or a mantra. This helps to still the mind and body, allowing us to connect with our innermost being. Through meditation, we come to understand that we are not our thoughts or emotions but that we are something much greater. We begin to see that we are limitless beings, existing beyond the confines of the physical world. As we connect with our true nature, we start to experience inner peace and happiness. We also become more compassionate and accepting of others. Kriya Yoga is a journey of self-discovery, and meditation is essential for making progress on this path.

2. Helps in Controlling Your Thoughts and Emotions

Kriya Yoga is an ancient practice that has been used for centuries to help people attain physical, mental, and spiritual enlightenment. One of the key aspects of Kriya Yoga is meditation. Meditation helps you control your thoughts and emotions, and it also allows you to connect with your higher self. When you meditate, you are able to quiet your mind and focus on your breath. This helps you slow down your thoughts, and it allows you to become more aware of your surroundings. As you become more aware of your thoughts and emotions, you are able to control them. This is essential in Kriya Yoga, as it allows you to focus on your spiritual journey and attain enlightenment.

3. Helps in Achieving a State of Inner Peace and Clarity

In Kriya Yoga, meditation is seen as an important tool in achieving a state of inner peace and clarity. The goal is to still the mind and achieve a state of union with the divine. In order to do this, practitioners must first learn to quiet their thoughts and focus their attention on their breath. Once the mind is calmed, practitioners can explore their inner consciousness. By meditating regularly, Kriya yogis eventually learn to control their thoughts and emotions, leading to a more peaceful and balanced state of mind. In addition to promoting mental wellbeing, meditation also has numerous physical benefits. It can help to lower blood pressure, improve cardiovascular health, and boost immunity. Moreover, meditation has been shown to increase dopamine and serotonin levels, two neurotransmitters known to promote feelings of happiness and wellbeing. Thus, it is clear that meditation plays an important role in Kriya Yoga and can be beneficial for both the body and the mind.

4. Helps You Develop a Stronger Connection to Your Higher Self

Kriya Yoga is a path of meditation and self-realization. The practice of Kriya Yoga leads to the union of the individual self with the infinite. In order to realize this union, it is essential to develop a strong connection with one's Higher Self. Meditation is a key component of Kriya Yoga, as it allows practitioners to go within and connect with their true nature. Through regular meditation, practitioners can develop a deep understanding of their own spiritual nature. Additionally, meditation helps to cleanse the mind and body of negative thoughts and emotions. As a result, meditation plays an important role in Kriya Yoga, as it helps practitioners to develop a stronger connection to their Higher Self. By establishing this connection, practitioners can begin to experience the true bliss of union with the infinite.

Kriya Meditation Techniques

1. Hong- Sau Technique

Meditation is a process of calming the mind and attaining inner peace. There are many different types of meditation, each with its own benefits. One type that can be particularly helpful in promoting relaxation and mental clarity is the Hong-Sau Technique. It is a form of Kriya meditation that is said to help practitioners connect with their higher selves. The practice involves focusing on the breath and using it to guide the movement of energy through the body. By channeling energy in this way, practitioners can access deeper levels of consciousness and connect with their true nature.

The Hong-Sau Technique is said to have many benefits, including improved concentration, reduced stress, and increased clarity of mind. The practice is also said to help practitioners develop a stronger connection with their higher selves, leading to a more fulfilling and meaningful life. This form of meditation involves focusing on the breath and mentally repeating the mantra "Hong Sau" with each inhale and "Sat Nam" with each exhale. The following steps can help you to get started:

1. To begin, find a comfortable place to sit or lie down. Close your eyes and take a few deep breaths, letting your body relax.
2. With your eyes closed, take a few deep breaths to center yourself. Once you feel relaxed, begin focusing on your breath.
3. Count each inhale and exhale. After a few breaths, start to mentally repeat the mantra "Hong Sau" with each inhale and "Sat Nam" with each exhale.
4. If your mind starts to wander, gently bring your attention back to your breath and the mantra. Continue for 10-20 minutes or longer if desired.
5. When you are finished, sit for a minute or two with your eyes closed and notice how you feel.

The Hong-Sau Technique is a form of meditation that is said to help practitioners focus and connect with their higher selves. The practice involves focusing on the breath and using a mantra to still the mind. While there are many different ways to meditate, this technique is a popular option for beginners as it is relatively simple and can be done anywhere.

2. Om Meditation Technique

Om meditation is a type of contemplation in which you focus your attention on the sound of the word "Om." The word "Om" is considered the most sacred sound in the universe and is believed to represent the divine energy that pervades all creation. Om is a sacred sound and symbol in Hinduism, Buddhism, Jainism, and Sikhism. It is also a popular Yoga and meditation chant. It is derived from the Sanskrit root Auṃ or Aum, and it represents the divine energy that pervades the universe. The sound of Om is said to be the sound of the universe itself. In Hinduism, Om is used as a mantra or sacred utterance, and it is often chanted at the beginning and end of Yoga sessions. It is also used as a greeting, farewell, and blessing. In Om meditation, you simply sit quietly and focus your mind on the sound of the word "Om." As you meditate, you may notice that your mind begins to quiet down and that you feel a sense of peace and calmness. You may also notice that your breathing becomes deeper and more regular. Aum meditation can be practiced for any length of time, but it is typically recommended to meditate for at least 20 minutes per day. With regular practice, you'll likely find that Om meditation helps to reduce stress, improve sleep, and increase feelings of wellbeing.

How to Perform Om Mantra Meditation

Step 1: The correct posture

The easiest way to perform Om meditation is to sit in a comfortable position with your spine straight. You can sit on the floor or in a chair, but make sure your back is not hunched over and your shoulders are relaxed. You may want to close your eyes or keep them open and focused on a spot on the ground in front of you.

Step 2: Focus on your breath

Once you're seated, take a few deep breaths and focus your attention on your breath. Feel the air fill your lungs as you inhale and then empty them as you exhale. If your mind starts to wander, simply bring your focus back to your breath.

Step 3: Repeat the mantra "Om"

After you've focused on your breathing for a few minutes, start repeating the mantra "Om." You can say it out loud or silently to yourself, but make sure that you enunciate each syllable clearly. Repeat the mantra as many times as you like, letting the sound flow naturally.

Step 4: Continue for as long as you like

You can continue repeating the mantra for as long as you like. If you find your mind wandering, simply bring your focus back to the sound of the mantra. When you're ready to stop, take a few deep breaths and slowly open your eyes.

3. Kundalini Kriya Meditation

Kundalini meditation is a type of mindfulness meditation that originated in India. The word "kundalini" comes from the Sanskrit word meaning "coiled up." This refers to the belief that there is a coiled-up energy at the base of the spine that can be awakened through Kundalini meditation. This form of meditation involves specific breathing exercises and mudras, or hand gestures, to stimulate the flow of energy along the spine. Kundalini is often described as a coiled snake that lies at the base of the spine, and the goal of this type of meditation is to awaken this energy and allow it to rise up through the chakras, or energy centers, of the body. Kundalini meditation can be used for a variety of purposes, including improving mental and physical health, developing psychic abilities, and enhancing spiritual growth.

The goal is to awaken this energy and bring it up through the body's chakras, or energy centers. This process is said to promote physical, mental, and emotional wellbeing. Kundalini meditation is often practiced with the help of a teacher or guru who can guide the practitioner through the process. While it can be beneficial to have some guidance when learning this type of meditation, it is not necessary. Anyone can learn how to practice Kundalini meditation by simply sitting quietly and focusing on their breath.

Steps:

> There are many different ways to practice Kundalini meditation, but one of the most popular methods is known as Sitali breath.
> 1. To begin, sit with your spine straight and your eyes closed. Take a deep breath through your nose, filling your lungs completely.

2. As you exhale, purse your lips and make a "ha" sound.
3. Continue breathing this way for several minutes.
4. You may also want to place your hands in a mudra known as Gyan mudra by touching your thumb and index finger together while keeping your other fingers extended. This mudra is said to promote concentration and wisdom.
5. As you continue to breathe deeply and rhythmically, allow your mind to become progressively more still.
6. If you find your thoughts wandering, gently bring them back to your breath.
7. Once you have achieved a state of deep relaxation, begin to focus on the sensation of energy at the base of your spine. Visualize this energy rising up through your chakras until it reaches the crown of your head.
8. Allow yourself to feel the blissful sensation of this energy coursing through your entire body. Remain in this state for as long as you like before slowly coming out of mediation.

4. Isha Kriya Meditation

Isha Kriya is a simple yet powerful process created by yogi and mystic, Sadhguru. It is designed to help you go beyond your body and mind and experience true inner peace. It is a guided meditation that can be done sitting in a chair with the spine straight or on the floor with the legs crossed. The practice includes specific instructions and predetermined movements designed to regulate one's breath and bring the body into a state of stillness. The goal of Isha Kriya is to help the individual move beyond the mind and experience the true nature of their being. While it is possible to do Isha Kriya on one's own, it is recommended that it be learned from a certified teacher. Once learned, it can be practiced daily and only takes 12-18 minutes to complete.

Steps:
1. The first step is to sit in a comfortable position with your spine erect. You can sit on the floor or in a chair. If you are sitting on the floor, you can cross your legs or sit in any other comfortable position.
2. Once you are seated comfortably, close your eyes and take a few deep breaths.

3. The next step is to focus your attention on the breath. Simply watch the breath as it comes in and out.
4. Do not try to control your breathing; just observe it. As you focus on it, you will notice that your mind will become quieter and still.
5. After a few minutes of focusing, begin the mantra isha by silently repeating the word "isha" with each inhalation and exhalation. The mantra isha means "the formless one." Repeating this mantra will help you to connect with the formless dimension within yourself.
6. Continue repeating the mantra isha for 11 minutes. Then, simply stay aware of your breath for a few minutes without repeating the mantra.
7. Finally, open your eyes and take a few deep breaths before getting up slowly from your seat.

5. Trataka Meditation

Trataka, also spelled *tratak,* is a yogic practice in which the meditator focuses on a single object, usually a candle flame, until tears run from the eyes. The practice is said to purify the nadi, or energetic channels of the body, and improve concentration. It is often practiced as part of a broader Yoga routine that includes asana (physical postures), pranayama (breath control), and meditation. The practice is said to improve concentration and mental clarity and alleviate stress and anxiety.

Steps:

1. Find a comfortable place to sit with your spine straight and your eyes open.
2. Fix your gaze on the object you have chosen, and do your best to maintain that gaze without blinking or looking away.
3. If your mind begins to wander, simply bring your attention back to the object.
4. You can start by doing trataka Kriya for five minutes at a time, gradually working up to longer sessions as you become more comfortable with the practice.
5. With regular practice, you'll begin to notice the benefits of trataka Kriya meditation in your everyday life.

There are two primary types of trataka, one with eyes open (aksha trataka) and the other with eyes closed (karna trataka). In aksha trataka, the meditator gazes at an object placed approximately two feet in front of them, typically a lit candle. The gaze should be steady and soft, without strain or blinking. If the eyes begin to water, they should be allowed to do so without wiping. After several minutes, the eyes are closed, and the object is visualized. This can be done for a minute or two before returning to the original gaze.

Karna trataka is similar to aksha trataka, but the object is placed slightly further away - about four feet - and looked at with closed eyes. In this case, it may be helpful to focus on the third eye point, or Ajna chakra, located between the eyebrows. As with aksha trataka, if tears appear, they should be allowed to flow freely. After some time, the image of the object may be visualized with closed eyes before returning to the original state.

Both types of trataka can be practiced for any length of time, though five minutes is generally considered a good place to start. With regular practice, it is said that one will develop greater concentration and clarity of mind, as well as improved vision and overall health.

Energization Technique

There are many energization techniques that can be done before and after meditation. A few examples are provided below.

Yoga

Yoga is a great way to prepare your body for meditation by stretching and loosening up the muscles. It can also help you relax and focus your mind. Meditation is a great way to relax and de-stress, but it can be difficult to keep your mind from wandering. One way to help focus your thoughts is to energize your body with some simple Yoga poses. Downward-facing dog, for example, is a great way to release tension from the back and neck. Child's pose is another good option for beginners, as it helps to stretch the hips and spine. Once you've completed a few basic poses, you'll be ready to sit down and clear your mind. By taking a few minutes to energize your body before meditation, you'll be able to focus more easily on the present moment.

Stretching

Stretching is another good way to loosen up the muscles and prepare your body for meditation. It is widely known that stretching before physical activity can prevent injuries. However, stretching can also be beneficial for those looking to improve their mental wellbeing. One of the most popular energization techniques that can be done before meditation is stretching. It increases blood flow and oxygen levels in the body, which can improve focus and concentration. In addition, stretching helps release muscle tension, improving relaxation during meditation. For best results, stretches should be performed slowly and smoothly, without jerking or bouncing movements. It is also important to listen to your body and only stretch to the point of mild discomfort. With regular practice, stretching can help you to achieve a deeper level of meditation and experience more benefits for your mind and body.

Guided Imagery

Guided imagery can be used to help you relax and focus your mind before and after meditation. Guided imagery is a visualization technique that can be used for various purposes, including relaxation, stress relief, and pain management. The idea behind guided imagery is that your mind is a powerful tool that can be harnessed to create positive change in your life. When you focus your thoughts on peaceful images or scenes, your brain begins to produce calming chemicals, such as endorphins and serotonin. This can lead to reduced stress levels and an overall feeling of wellbeing. Guided imagery can be done either with the help of a therapist or on your own at home. If you decide to do it on your own, there are a few things that you should keep in mind. First, it's important to find a comfortable place to sit or lie down. Close your eyes and take several deep breaths to help you relax. Once you're feeling calm, begin to imagine a peaceful scene. It can be anything from a quiet meadow to a secluded beach. Visualize every detail of the scene, from the colors and smells to the textures and sounds. Allow yourself to spend some time exploring the scene before slowly coming back to the present moment. When you're finished, take a few deep breaths and open your eyes. Guided imagery is a simple but effective way to reduce stress and promote relaxation.

Breathing Exercises

Breathing exercises can help you relax and focus your mind before and after meditation. Energization techniques are a great way to get yourself moving post-meditation. Specifically, breathing exercises can help to increase your energy levels and focus. The first step is to take a deep breath through your nose. As you inhale, feel your stomach expand. Then, exhale slowly through your mouth. Repeat this process for a few minutes. You should feel your energy level rising with each breath. In addition, try to focus on a positive thought or image with each inhale and exhale. This will further increase your energy and focus.

Chapter 8: Asanas: Kriya Poses to Master

Asanas are one of the key components of Kriya Yoga, a spiritual practice focused on cleansing the body and mind to open oneself up to higher levels of awareness. Several different asanas can be used in kriya, each with its own set of benefits and challenges. Some of the most common asanas include inversions, backbends, balances, and twists. Each type of asana stimulates a different part of the body and mind, providing specific mental and physical benefits along with an insight into one's self.

Whether you're just starting with kriya or have been practicing for years, incorporating asanas into your routine will help you grow spiritually and physically. With consistent practice, you may find that your entire outlook on life begins to shift for the better. This chapter will provide instructions on performing some of the most common and beneficial asanas used in Kriya Yoga. It'll cover everything from the all-important sun salutation to more advanced inversions and twists. By the end, you'll have a strong foundation on which to build your kriya practice.

1. Fish Pose (Meenasana)

Known as the fish pose, Meenasana is a highly effective Yoga pose that is commonly used to improve flexibility and release tension in the body. To perform this pose, you first need to lie down on your back with your legs stretched out and your arms resting at your sides. Bend both legs at the knees and gently drop one knee to the side of your body and allow it to rest just above the floor. You then repeat this motion with the other leg so that both knees are on either side of your body. Finally, slowly lower the upper half of your body down onto the floor, allowing it to rest just slightly above your thighs or lower hips while keeping your shoulders aligned directly over your pelvis.

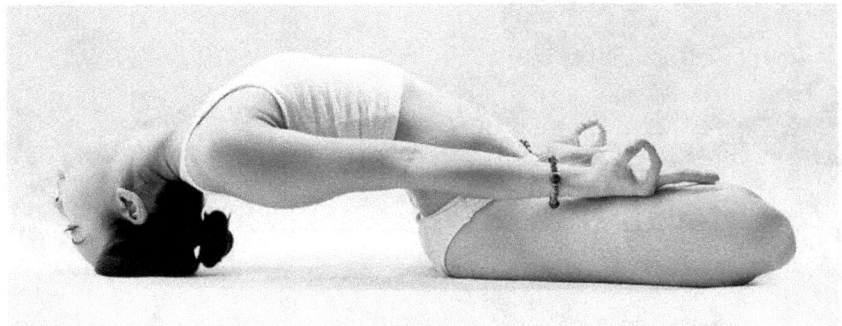

Fish pose.
Mr. Yoga, CC BY-SA 4.0 <https://creativecommons.org/licenses/by-sa/4.0>, via Wikimedia Commons https://commons.wikimedia.org/wiki/File:Mr-yoga-fish-pose.jpg

Maintaining this position for several breaths will help to lengthen and stretch all of the muscles along the sides of your body and promote overall relaxation. Due to its many benefits, the fish pose has become a go-to Yoga pose for people looking for stress relief and better flexibility. If you're looking for a way to relax after a long day or boost mobility in those tight spots, try the fish pose!

2. Cobra Pose (Pambu Asana)

Cobra Pose, also known as Pambu Asana, is a dynamic and invigorating Yoga posture that works both the upper and lower body. This pose engages the back muscles, particularly the erector spinae, enhancing core strength and improving overall posture. For this reason, this pose is often recommended if you're dealing with back pain and stiffness. In addition to its therapeutic benefits, Cobra Pose also helps strengthen your glutes and quads, improving stability in these key body regions.

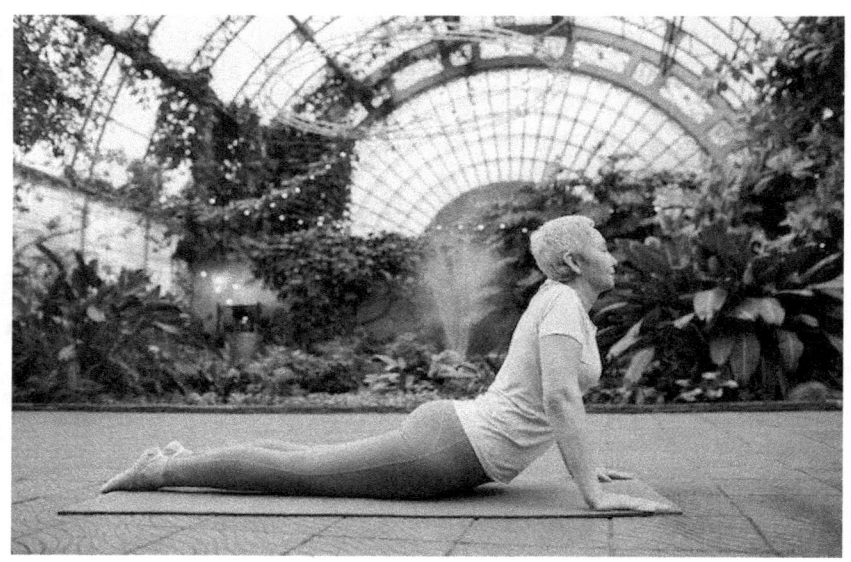

Cobra pose.
https://www.pexels.com/photo/woman-doing-cobra-pose-6787216/

To perform this pose, lie flat on your stomach with your legs extended behind you and your palms placed flat on the floor beside your chest. As you inhale, press down through your palms and begin to straighten your arms, lifting your torso and lower body off of the ground. Keep your shoulders pulled back and down away from your ears as you continue to lift your chest higher. Gaze upwards, taking care not to strain your neck. Hold this pose for 5-10 breaths before slowly lowering back down to the starting position.

As you hold this pose, you'll feel the energy coursing through your entire body, leaving you feeling refreshed and revitalized. Whether you are an experienced yogi or a beginner, give Cobra Pose a try – you'll be amazed by its many benefits!

3. Seated Crane Pose (Amaranth Kokuasana)

Seated Crane Pose, also known as Amaranth Kokuasana, is a Yoga pose that focuses primarily on strength and flexibility. In this pose, you begin by sitting upright with your legs fully extended in front of you. Then, slowly bend your knees and bring your feet in towards your body, pressing the soles of your feet together and gently drawing them upward until they are at a 90-degree angle to your body. Next, using the strength of your arms and core, you lower yourself down so that your back is flat on the floor and hold this position for several deep breaths. Seated Crane Pose helps improve balance, build muscles in the arms and legs, and stretch out key body parts.

4. Sun Salutation (Surya Namaskar)

Sun Salutation, also known as Surya Namaskar, is a staple of many Yoga practices. This sequence is designed to bring energy and vitality into every part of the body, awakening the mind and spirit along the way. The actual movements involved in Sun Salutation are simple yet powerful, helping to stretch and strengthen muscles while also promoting better circulation and alignment. Additionally, this practice is believed to stimulate the body's chakras and other energetic centers, leaving us feeling refreshed, balanced, and renewed.

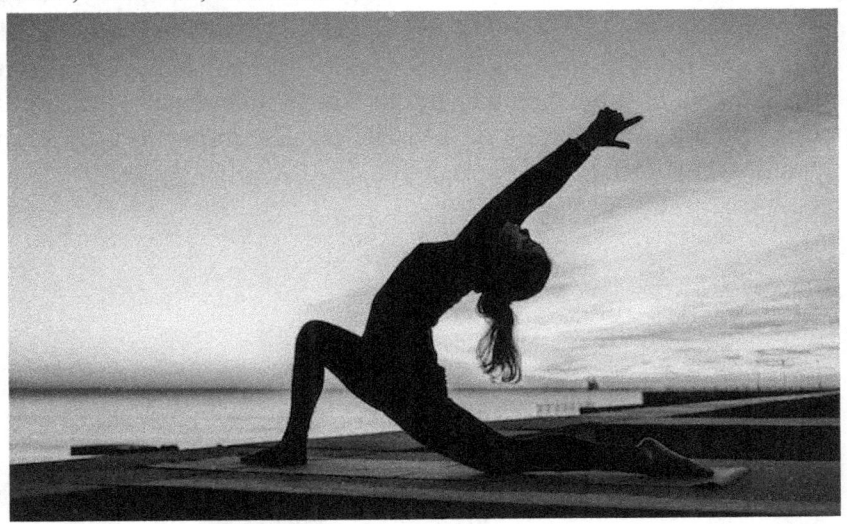

Sun salutation.
https://unsplash.com/photos/F2qh3yjz6Jk

To perform Sun Salutation, you begin in a standing position with your feet together and your hands at your sides. From here, you inhale as you raise your arms overhead, then exhale as you bend forward from the waist and place your palms flat on the floor beside your feet. Inhaling once again, lift your head and chest up off the floor and arch your back, looking up toward the sky. Exhaling deeply, you return to the forward bend position.

Continuing to move with your breath, you inhale as you step your right foot back into a low lunge, then exhale as you bring your left foot back to meet it in the plank position. From here, lower your entire body down to the floor, keeping your elbows close to your sides and your gaze fixed on the floor between your hands. Inhaling deeply, you press up into Upward Facing Dog, then exhale as you return to the plank position. Finally, you inhale as you step your right foot forward to meet your left, then exhale as you return to standing.

Sun Salutation is a versatile practice that can be performed at any time of day, making it an ideal way to start your morning or wind down before bed. Give it a try - you'll love the way it makes you feel!

5. Camel Pose (Ustrasana)

Camel Pose, also known as Ustrasana, is a powerful backbend that can help to open and strengthen the entire body. This pose begins in a kneeling position with your hands placed on top of your lower back, directly over your hips. As you slowly lean back and stretch your chest toward the sky, be sure to keep your knees and thighs flat on the ground. This challenging posture can feel intense at first, but with practice and proper alignment, it can have a profoundly positive impact on the strength and flexibility of your back and spine.

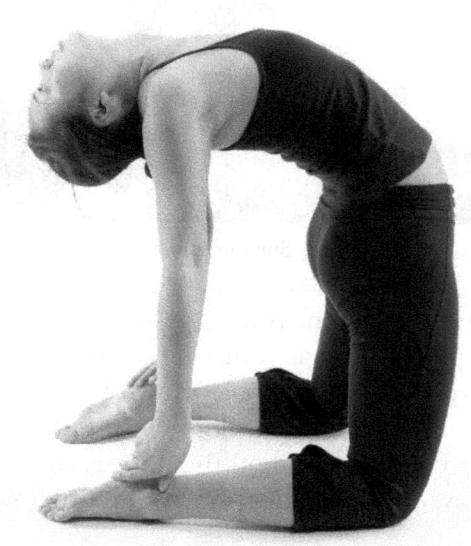

Camel pose.
lululemon athletica, CC BY 2.0 <https://creativecommons.org/licenses/by/2.0>, via Wikimedia Commons https://commons.wikimedia.org/wiki/File:Ustrasana_-_Camel_Pose.jpg

The advantages of Camel Pose are many. It improves posture and alleviates back, neck, and shoulder pain. Additionally, it can help to boost energy levels and increase circulation throughout the body. Camel Pose is also believed to stimulate the thyroid gland and promote emotional balance. If you're looking for a powerful way to open and strengthen your body from head to toe, give Camel Pose a try!

6. Cow Face Pose (Bitilasana)

Cow Face Pose, also known as Bitilasana, is a gentle Yoga position that is recommended for all levels of practitioners. It is designed to stretch and open the chest and shoulders, helping to increase lung capacity and relieve tension in the upper body. Many people also find that this pose improves focus and concentration, making it a great choice for students or professionals who need to stay sharp and focused.

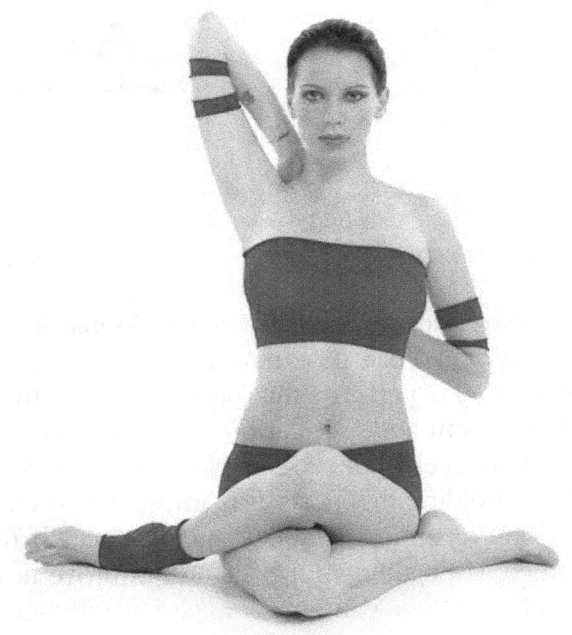

Cow face pose.
Kennguru, CC BY 3.0 <https://creativecommons.org/licenses/by/3.0>, via Wikimedia Commons
https://commons.wikimedia.org/wiki/File:Gomukhasana_Yoga-Asana_Nina-Mel.jpg

To perform Cow Face Pose, begin by sitting on your mat with your legs folded in front of you. Keeping your back straight and your gaze forward, bring your right arm up so that the right hand meets the left elbow. Slowly breathe deeply as you hold this position for at least one minute. To release, simply switch sides and repeat. With practice, Cow Face Pose can become a powerful tool for boosting energy and relieving stress. Why not give it a try today? You just might be surprised by how good it makes you feel!

7. Bridge Pose (Setubandha Asana)

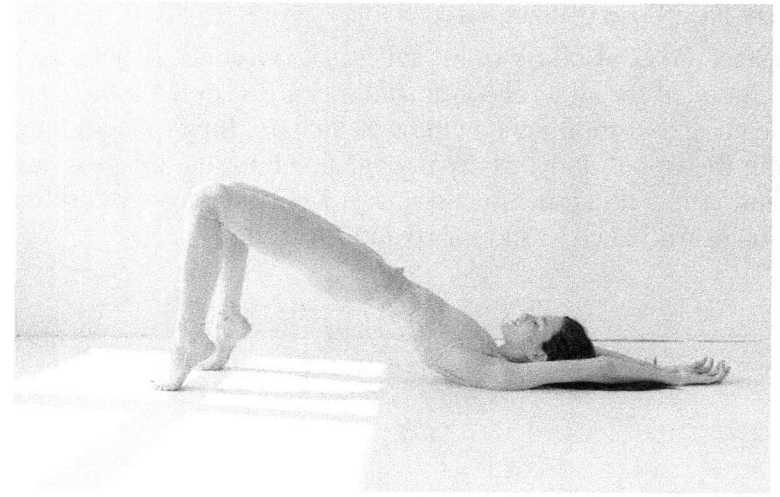

Bridge pose.
https://www.pexels.com/photo/graceful-woman-performing-variation-of-setu-bandha-sarvangasana-yoga-pose-5012071/

Bridge Pose, also known as Setubandha Asana in Sanskrit, is a challenging but rewarding Yoga pose that targets the deep muscles of the back, sides, and core. To perform this pose, you start by lying on your back with your knees bent and feet flat on the floor. Then, you slowly lift your hips until you feel that your spine is fully lengthened and straightened. While holding this pose, it is important to engage all of the core muscles to achieve optimal stability and balance. If done correctly, Bridge Pose can help strengthen your back and improve flexibility in your hips and shoulders. Whether you are an experienced yogi or just starting on your journey toward wellness, don't forget to include Bridge Pose in your practice!

8. Thunderbolt Pose (Vajrasana)

Thunderbolt Pose, also known as Vajrasana, is a powerful Yoga pose that has many benefits for the body and mind. This kneeling posture deeply stretches the hips and thighs, making it an ideal choice for anyone who spends a lot of time sitting or running. Furthermore, Thunderbolt

Pose helps strengthen and tone the lower body muscles, improving balance and coordination. In addition, this pose has been shown to have mental benefits as well, improving concentration and helping to boost mood.

To perform the Thunderbolt Pose, begin by sitting on your heels with your knees wide apart. Then, place your hands on the floor in front of you and slowly lean back until you feel a stretch in your thighs and hips. Be sure to keep your back straight and your gaze forward as you hold this pose for at least one minute. To release, simply come back to a sitting position and repeat on the other side. With regular practice, Thunderbolt Pose can help to improve your flexibility, stamina, and overall sense of wellbeing.

9. Corpse Pose (Savasana)

The Corpse Pose, or savasana, is an essential part of any Yoga practice. This calming and restorative pose relaxes your body and mind during intense physical activity, allowing you to fully let go and reconnect with your inner self. When done correctly, the Corpse Pose can help stretch and realign the spine, releasing tension from the back and shoulders. It also promotes deep breathing and improves circulation throughout the body.

To perform the Corpse Pose, simply lie on your back with your legs and arms extended. Make sure that your feet are about hip-width apart and your palms are facing up. Then, close your eyes and focus on your breath. Allow your whole body to relax and sink into the mat. Stay in this position for at least five minutes or longer. Whether you are a seasoned yogi or just getting started with your practice, this simple yet powerful pose will leave you feeling refreshed, grounded, and renewed. Take some time today to lay back, breathe deeply, and try out the corpse pose for yourself! You won't regret it.

10. Lion Pose (Simhasana)

Lion Pose, also known as simhasana, is a Yoga pose that is often used as part of a meditation or deep breathing practice. This pose gets its name from how it mimics the powerful and noble stance of the lion. To practice this pose, you first need to sit on the floor with your legs crossed and your back straight. Then, you'll slowly force your tongue out of your mouth until it touches the underside of your chin. As you hold this position, you may notice that it helps to open up and release tension throughout your face and neck. Additionally, many people find that strength training their facial muscles through this pose can help to ease symptoms associated with TMJ disorder and other similar conditions. Overall, the Lion Pose can be a great way to loosen up and relax after a long day.

11. Head to Knee Pose (Janu Sirsasana)

Head-to-knee Pose, or Janu sirsasana, is a classic Yoga pose that is often used in vinyasa and Hatha classes. This pose can offer several benefits, from stretching the hamstrings and the lower back to helping to improve balance and focus. To begin, start by sitting on the floor with your legs extended straight out in front of you. Take one leg and bend it up towards your body, bringing your foot towards your crotch. If possible, try to bring the sole of your foot as close to your navel as possible. Once your leg is in position, slowly reach down and take hold of either side of your foot with both hands. Then slowly start to lengthen through the spine while simultaneously exhaling and rounding over the extended leg. Hold this position for several deep breaths before switching sides. With regular practice, the head-to-knee pose can offer many physical and mental benefits that make it well worth adding to any Yoga practice.

12. Triangle Pose (Trikonasana)

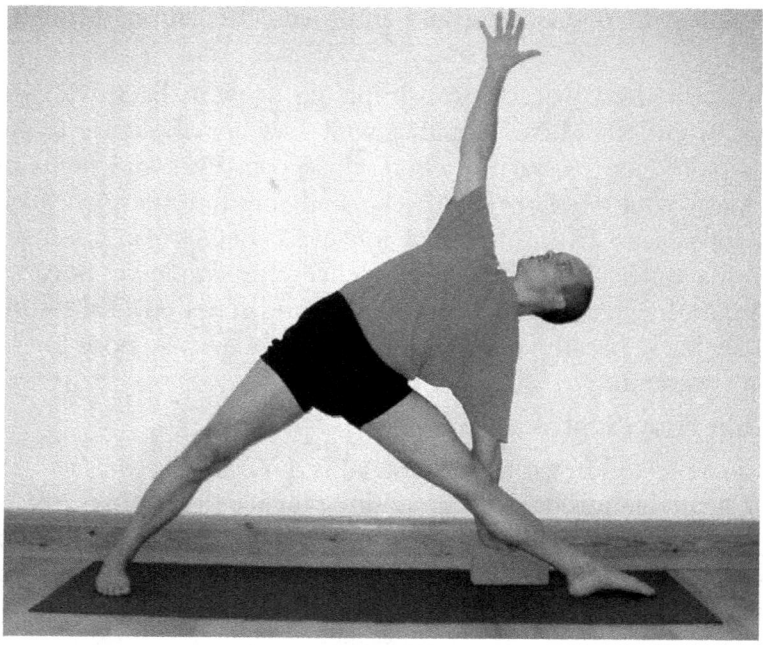

Triangle pose.
Matthew Greenfield, CC BY-SA 3.0 <https://creativecommons.org/licenses/by-sa/3.0>, via Wikimedia Commons https://commons.wikimedia.org/wiki/File:Uttitha_Trikonasana.jpg

Triangle Pose, or trikonasana, is one of the basic Yoga poses widely practiced in many types of Yoga and wellness regimes. This pose requires you to stand with your legs far apart, your toes pointed forward, and your heels slightly inward. Then, reach out to the sides, pivot at the pelvis, and extend your arms straight up into the air. The Triangle Pose is particularly excellent for opening up the hips and helping you to feel more balanced and centered. It also stimulates circulation throughout your body and can help to stretch and tone the muscles of your legs and arms. Overall, the Triangle Pose is a great way for anyone looking for an effective and introspective practice that can enhance flexibility, strength, and focus.

13. Half Spinal Twist Pose (Ardha Matsyendrasana)

The Half Spinal Twist Pose, or Ardha Matsyendrasana, is a staple of many Yoga classes. To perform this pose, you'll need to start by sitting on the floor with your legs extended out in front of you. Then, take your right leg and bend it up so that your foot is resting flat against your left thigh. Next, twist your torso to the right and reach your left arm around the outside of your right knee. Finally, complete the pose by reaching your right arm around behind you and grabbing hold of your left hamstring. The Half Spinal Twist Pose is a great way to stretch the muscles of your back and shoulders, as well as stimulate circulation throughout your body.

This powerful twist opens up the hips and stretches out the lower back, making it perfect for both beginners and seasoned yogis alike. Additionally, this pose counteracts the negative effects of prolonged sitting by gently loosening tight muscles and joints. For these reasons, regularly practicing the Half Spinal Twist Pose is a great way to help promote healthy body alignment and prevent chronic musculoskeletal pain.

14. Child Pose (Shishu Asana)

Child Pose is a popular Yoga asana that is often used to calm and rejuvenate the body. To begin, start by sitting on your heels with your knees bent and your feet flat against the floor. Then, slowly lean forward and place your forehead on the mat in front of you. Next, extend your arms out in front of you and allow your chest and torso to relax down onto your thighs. Finally, take several deep breaths and focus on relaxing your entire body. The Child Pose is an excellent way to stretch out the back and shoulder muscles and help improve circulation throughout the body.

Additionally, this pose can help reduce stress and anxiety, making it perfect for anyone looking for a way to unwind and relax. This comfortable position also stretches and relaxes the hips, spine, and neck while also promoting deep breathing. Some people even believe that practicing Child Pose regularly can help reduce stress and anxiety, making this asana a great option for those looking to quickly escape everyday pressures.

15. Seated Forward Bend (Paschimottanasana)

At first glance, the seated forward bend might seem like a simple exercise. However, this pose offers a wide range of benefits for both the mind and body. For starters, a seated forward bend stretches out the hamstrings, calves, and hips, helping to improve flexibility and relieve muscle tension. It also increases blood flow to the brain and helps to stimulate the glands in the neck, shoulder blades, and spine. On a mental level, this pose can help calm your mind and reduce stress or anxiety.

To perform a seated forward bend, start by sitting on the floor with your legs extended out in front of you. Next, reach your arms up overhead and then slowly lean forward from the hips, reaching your hands toward your feet. If you can't quite reach your toes, don't worry; simply place your hands wherever they comfortably fall. Once you are in the forward bend, take several deep breaths and focus on relaxing your entire body. Remember to keep your spine straight and your shoulders relaxed as you hold the pose. To release the pose, slowly roll back up to a seated position and take a few deep breaths before moving on to the next asana.

There are many different Yoga asanas or poses that offer a variety of benefits for both the mind and body. In this chapter, we have presented 15 different Yoga asanas that are perfect for beginners. Each asana has its specific purpose and advantages, so be sure to choose the poses that best suit your needs. Remember to focus on your breath and relaxation as you move through each pose, and always consult with a doctor before beginning any new exercise routine. With regular practice, you will notice an improvement in your flexibility, muscle strength, and overall sense of wellbeing.

Chapter 9: Kriya Yoga Sequences: Putting It All Together

Now that you're familiar with the various poses, mudras, mantras, and breathing patterns used in Kriya yoga, it's time to put them all together into full sequences. These can be done every day of the week or any day you're free. Remember to warm up before each sequence with simple stretches and cool down afterward with restorative poses. Most importantly, listen to your body and don't push yourself too hard – Kriya yoga should be enjoyable, not torturous. This chapter will give you seven complete Kriya yoga sequences, one for each day of the week. These sequences are meant to give you a starting point from which you can create your own. If you're just starting out, though, you can use the following sequences as-is.

Monday Routine

Monday's routine is a gentle one designed to ease you into the week. It begins with some basic standing poses to get your energy flowing, then moves into a simple forward fold and some twists to release any tension you may be holding in your body. The sequence ends with some restorative poses to help you relax and reset for the week ahead.

Poses
1. **Tadasana (Mountain Pose):** Stand with your feet together, arms by your sides. Take a deep breath in and raise your arms overhead, then exhale and fold forward, bringing your hands

to the floor.
2. **Uttanasana (Standing Forward Fold):** From Tadasana, exhale and fold forward, bringing your hands to the floor. If you can't reach the floor, place your hands on your shins or a block.
3. **Ardha Uttanasana (Half Lift Pose):** From Uttanasana, place your hands on your hips and inhale as you lift your chest and torso halfway up.
4. **Parivritta Trikonasana (Revolved Triangle Pose):** From Ardha Uttanasana, step your left foot back and exhale as you rotate your torso to the right, bringing your right hand to the floor and your left arm toward the ceiling. Repeat on the other side.
5. **Pasasana (Noose Pose):** From Parivritta Trikonasana, take your left hand to the floor and your right hand to your left ankle, then exhale as you twist your torso to the left. Repeat on the other side.

Mantras
1. **Om Namo Narayanaya (Vishnu Mantra):** Chant this mantra 108 times while in Pasasana.
2. **Om Shri Durgayai Namah (Durga Mantra):** Chant this mantra 108 times while in Ardha Uttanasana.

Mudras
1. **Gyan Mudrā:** Sit in a comfortable position with your spine straight. Bring your index finger and thumb together, then rest your other three fingers lightly on your palm.
2. **Pranava Mudrā:** Sit in a comfortable position with your spine straight. Bring your index finger and middle finger to touch at the tips, then press your thumb against your palm.
3. **Apana Mudrā:** Sit in a comfortable position with your spine straight. Press your ring finger and little finger into your palm, then touch the tips of your thumb and index finger together.

Breath Pattern: Ujjayi Breathing

To do Ujjayi breathing, simply breathe deeply and steadily through your nose, expanding your belly as you inhale and contracting it as you exhale. As you exhale, close your throat slightly and make an "ahh" sound. You should feel slight resistance in your throat as if you were fogging up a mirror.

Closing Poses
1. Viparita Karani (Legs-Up-the-Wall Pose): Lie on your back with your legs against a wall and your arms by your sides.
2. Savasana (Corpse Pose): From Viparita Karani, let your legs fall to one side and your arms fall to the other, then simply allow your whole body to relax and sink into the floor.
3. Namaste: Sit in a comfortable position with your spine straight. Bring your palms together in front of your chest and bow your head, then say "Namaste" either aloud or silently to yourself.

Tuesday Routine

This routine is designed to get your blood flowing and your energy up. It begins with some basic standing poses and moves into a more active flow, including some sun salutations. The sequence ends with a few calming postures to help you wind down before bed.

Poses
1. **Surya Namaskar (Sun Salutation) A:** Stand with your feet together and your arms by your sides. Inhale as you raise your arms overhead, then exhale as you fold forward and place your hands on the floor.
2. **Paschimottanasana (Seated Forward Fold):** From Surya Namaskar A, exhale and bring your chin to your chest, then fold forward and place your hands on the floor.
3. **Bhujangasana (Cobra Pose):** From Paschimottanasana, place your hands on the floor beside you and inhale as you lift your chest and head off the floor.
4. **Adho Mukha Svanasana (Downward-Facing Dog Pose):** From Bhujangasana, exhale and lift your hips up and back, straightening your legs and pressing your heels into the floor.
5. **Janu Sirsasana (Head-to-Knee Pose):** From Downward-Facing Dog, inhale and take your right leg forward, then exhale and fold forward, placing your forehead on your right knee.

Mantras
1. **Om Namo Bhagavate Vasudevaya (Vishnu Mantra):** Chant this mantra 108 times while in Paschimottanasana.

2. **Om Shri Krishna Sharanam Mama (Krishna Mantra):** Chant this mantra 108 times while in Bhujangasana.

Mudras

1. **Prithvi Mudrā:** Sit in a comfortable position with your spine straight. Place your palms on the floor beside you, then press your thumbs and index fingers together.
2. **Jnana Mudrā:** Sit in a comfortable position with your spine straight. Bend your index finger and middle finger to touch your palm, then press your thumb against your palm.
3. **Shuni Mudrā:** Sit in a comfortable position with your spine straight. Bend your ring finger and little finger to touch your palm, then press your thumb against your palm.

Breath Pattern: Sama Vritti Breathing

To do Sama Vritti breathing, simply breathe steadily through your nose, making sure that your inhales and exhales are of equal duration.

Closing Poses

1. **Balasana (Child's Pose):** From Downward-Facing Dog, exhale and lower your hips to your heels, then rest your forehead on the floor.
2. **Viparita Karani (Legs-Up-the-Wall Pose):** Lie on your back with your legs against a wall and your arms by your sides.
3. **Savasana (Corpse Pose):** From Viparita Karani, let your legs fall to one side and your arms fall to the other, then simply let your whole body relax and sink into the floor.
4. **Namaste:** Sit in a comfortable position with your spine straight. Bring your palms together in front of your chest and bow your head, then say "Namaste" aloud or silently.

Wednesday Routine

This routine is designed to help you focus and center yourself. It begins with some basic standing and seated poses, then moves into a series of twists to help release any tension in your spine. The sequence ends with a few calming postures to help you wind down before bed.

Poses

1. **Virabhadrasana I (Warrior I Pose):** From Tadasana, put your left foot back and raise your arms overhead, then lunge

forward with your right leg.
2. **Parivrtta Trikonasana (Revolved Triangle Pose):** From the Warrior pose, bring your left hand to the floor inside your left foot, then twist your torso to the left and reach your right arm up toward the ceiling.
3. **Ardha Matsyendrasana (Half Lord of the Fishes Pose):** Sit on the floor with your legs straight in front of you, then bend your right knee and place your right foot outside your left thigh. Twist your torso to the right and place your left elbow outside your right knee, then reach your right arm behind you and place your hand on the floor.

Mantras
1. **Om Mantra:** Chant this mantra 108 times while in Warrior I Pose.
2. **Gayatri Mantra:** Chant this mantra 108 times while in Revolved Triangle Pose.
3. **Maha Mrityunjaya Mantra:** Chant this mantra 108 times while in Half Lord of the Fishes Pose.

Mudras
1. **Anjali Mudra:** Sit in a comfortable position with your spine straight. Bring your palms together in front of your chest and bow your head.
2. **Hridaya Mudra:** Sit in a comfortable position with your spine straight. Place your right palm on your heart, then place your left palm over it.
3. **Shanmukhi Mudra:** Sit in a comfortable position with your spine straight. Touch the tips of your thumb, index finger, and middle finger together, then place your ring finger and little finger on the floor.

Breath Pattern: Sitali Breathing

To do Sitali breathing, curl your tongue into a "U" shape and stick it out of your mouth. Inhale through your mouth, then exhale through your nose.

Closing Poses
1. **Supta Baddha Konasana (Reclining Bound Angle Pose):** Lie on your back with your knees bent and your feet together, then

let your knees fall open to the sides.
2. **Viparita Karani (Legs-Up-the-Wall Pose):** Lie on your back with your legs against a wall and your arms by your sides.
3. **Savasana (Corpse Pose):** From Viparita Karani, let your legs fall to one side and your arms fall to the other, then simply let your whole body relax and sink into the floor.

Thursday Routine

This routine is designed to help you increase your flexibility. It begins with some basic standing and seated poses, then moves into a series of deeper stretches for your hips, hamstrings, and shoulders. The sequence ends with a few calming postures to help you wind down before bed.

Poses
1. **Bhujangasana (Cobra Pose):** Lie on your stomach with your legs straight and your hands by your sides, then press up into an upward-facing dog pose.
2. **Salabhasana (Locust Pose):** Lie on your stomach with your legs straight and your hands by your sides, then lift your chest and legs off the floor.
3. **Dhanurasana (Bow Pose):** Lie on your stomach with your legs straight and your hands by your sides, then reach back and grab your ankles.

Mantras
1. **Om Aim Hreem Kleem Chamundaye Vichche (Durga Mantra):** Chant this mantra 108 times while in Cobra Pose.
2. **Om Namo Bhagavate Vasudevaya (Vishnu Mantra):** Chant this mantra 108 times while in Locust Pose.

Mudras
1. **Prana Mudra:** Sit in a comfortable position with your spine straight. Raise your hands in front of you with your palms facing each other, then touch your thumbs to your index fingers.
2. **Samudra Mudra:** Sit in a comfortable position with your spine straight. Raise your hands in front of you with your palms facing each other, then touch your thumbs to your middle fingers.

3. **Hakini Mudra:** Sit in a comfortable position with your spine straight. Place your hands on your thighs with your palms facing up, then touch the tips of your thumb, index finger, and middle finger together.

Breath Pattern: Bhastrika Breathing

To do Bhastrika breathing, inhale and exhale rapidly through your nose. The breath should be deep and forceful but not so much so that you feel dizzy or lightheaded.

Closing Poses

1. **Paschimottanasana (Seated Forward Bend):** Sit on the floor with your legs straight in front of you, then lean forward and reach for your toes.
2. **Halasana (Plow Pose):** Lie on your back with your legs straight, then lift your hips and legs off the floor and over your head.
3. **Sarvangasana (Shoulder Stand):** Lie on your back with your legs straight and your arms by your sides, then lift your hips and legs off the floor and over your head.
4. **Matsyasana (Fish Pose):** Lie on your back with your legs straight and your arms by your sides, then lift your chest and head off the floor.
5. **Savasana (Corpse Pose):** From Matsyasana, let your legs fall to one side and your arms fall to the other, then simply let your whole body relax and sink into the floor.

Friday Routine

This routine is designed to help you increase your strength and stamina. It begins with some basic standing and seated poses, then moves into a series of more challenging postures that will test your endurance. The sequence ends with a few calming postures to help you wind down before bed.

Poses

1. **Adho Mukha Svanasana (Downward-Facing Dog Pose):** Start in a tabletop position with your hands and knees on the floor, then lift your hips and straighten your legs to form an upside-down "V" shape.
2. **Urdhva Mukha Svanasana (Upward-Facing Dog Pose):** Start in a downward-facing dog pose, then lift your chest and head off

the floor and press back into an upward-facing dog pose.
3. **Bakasana (Crane Pose):** Start in a tabletop position with your hands and knees on the floor, then lift your hips and straighten your legs to form an upside-down "V" shape.
4. **Salabhasana (Locust Pose):** Lie on your stomach with your legs straight and your hands by your sides, then lift your chest and legs off the floor.
5. **Dhanurasana (Bow Pose):** Lie on your stomach with your legs straight and your hands by your sides, then reach back and grab your ankles.

Mantras
1. **Om Aim Hreem Kleem Chamundaye Vichche (Durga Mantra):** Chant this mantra 108 times while in Cobra Pose.
2. **Om Namo Bhagavate Vasudevaya (Vishnu Mantra):** Chant this mantra 108 times while in Locust Pose.

Mudras
1. **Abhaya Mudra:** Sit in a comfortable position with your spine straight. Raise your right hand in front of you with your palm facing out, then touch your thumb to your index finger.
2. **Varada Mudra:** Sit in a comfortable position with your spine straight. Raise your right hand in front of you with your palm facing out, then touch your thumb to your middle finger.
3. **Vayu Mudra:** Sit in a comfortable position with your spine straight. Raise your right hand in front of you with the thumb and index finger touching each other, then touch the tips of your ring finger and little finger to your palm.
4. **Prithvi Mudra:** Sit in a comfortable position with your spine straight. Raise your right hand in front of you with the thumb and index finger touching each other, then touch the tip of your middle finger to the base of your thumb.
5. **Akasha Mudra:** Sit in a comfortable position with your spine straight. Raise your right hand in front of you with the thumb and index finger touching each other, then touch the tip of your ring finger and little finger to your palm.

Breath Pattern: Kapalabhati (Skull Shining Breath)

To practice this breath, sit in a comfortable position with your spine straight. Place your hands on your knees with your palms facing up. Breathe in and out through your nose; as you breathe out, contract your abdominal muscles so that your stomach pushes down and in. Do this rapidly for 10 breaths, then relax and breathe normally.

Saturday Routine

This routine is designed to help your flexibility and improve your balance. It begins with some basic standing and seated poses, then moves into a series of more challenging postures that will test your balance and flexibility. The sequence ends with a few calming postures to help you wind down before bed.

Poses
1. **Balasana (Child's Pose):** Start in a tabletop position with your hands and knees on the floor, then sit back on your heels and lower your forehead to the floor.
2. **Supta Baddha Konasana (Reclining Bound Angle Pose):** Lie on your back with your knees bent and your feet together, then allow your knees to fall open to the sides.
3. **Setu Bandha Sarvangasana (Bridge Pose):** Lie on your back with your knees bent and your feet flat on the floor, then lift your hips and chest off the floor and press your feet into the floor.
4. **Ardha Chandrasana (Half Moon Pose):** Start in a Warrior III pose, then reach your arms out to the sides and bend your torso to the right, reaching your left hand to the floor.

Mantras
1. **Om Shri Durgayai Namah (Durga Mantra):** Chant this mantra 108 times while in Child's Pose.
2. **Om Namo Bhagavate Vasudevaya (Vishnu Mantra):** Chant this mantra 108 times while in Reclining Bound Angle Pose.

Mudras
1. **Akasha Mudra:** Sit in a comfortable position with your spine straight. Raise your right hand in front of you with the thumb and index finger touching each other, then touch the tip of

your ring finger and little finger to your palm.
2. **Prithvi Mudra:** Sit in a comfortable position with your spine straight. Raise your right hand in front of you with the thumb and index finger touching each other, then touch the tip of your middle finger to the base of your thumb.
3. **Vayu Mudra:** Sit in a comfortable position with your spine straight. Raise your right hand in front of you with the thumb and index finger touching each other, then touch the tips of your ring finger and little finger to your palm.

Breath Pattern: Alternate Nostril Breathing (Nadi Shodhana)

To practice this breath, sit in a comfortable position with your spine straight. Close your right nostril with your right thumb and inhale through your left nostril. Then close your left nostril with your right ring and little fingers and exhale through your right nostril. Continue alternating nostrils, inhaling and exhaling through each one in turn. Do this for 10 breaths, then release the hand mudras and breathe normally.

Sunday Routine

This routine is designed to help you relax and unwind after a busy week. It begins with some basic standing and seated poses, then moves into a series of more restorative postures that will help your body and mind to relax.

Poses
1. **Halasana (Plow Pose):** Lie on your back with your legs straight, then lift your hips and legs off the floor and over your head.
2. **Karnapidasana (Ear Pressure Pose):** Lie on your back with your knees bent and your feet flat on the floor, then lift your hips and chest off the floor and press your palms into your ears.
3. **Supta Matsyendrasana (Supine Spinal Twist Pose):** Lie on your back with your legs straight, then lift your right leg and place it over your left leg. Reach your right arm out to the side and place it on the floor, then twist your torso to the left.

Mantras
1. **Om Namah Shivaya (Shiva Mantra):** Chant this mantra 108 times while in Plow Pose.

2. **Om Namo Narayanaya (Narayana Mantra):** Chant this mantra 108 times while in Ear Pressure Pose.

Mudras

1. **Jalandhara Mudra:** Sit in a comfortable position with your spine straight. Lower your chin down to your chest and place your palms on the floor beside you, then press your palms into the floor and lift your chin to the ceiling.
2. **Mula Bandha Mudra:** Sit in a comfortable position with your spine straight. Press your palms into the floor beside you, then lift your hips off the floor and clasp your ankles with your hands.
3. **Uddīyāna Bandha Mudra:** Sit in a comfortable position with your spine straight. Bend your knees and place your palms on the floor beside you, then press your palms into the floor and lift your hips off the floor. Clasp your ankles with your hands and arch your back.

Breath Pattern: 4-7-8 Breathing (Pranayama)

To practice this breath pattern, sit in a comfortable position with your spine straight. Place your hands on your stomach and inhale deeply through your nose, then exhale through your mouth while making a whooshing sound. Repeat this breath pattern for 4 minutes.

Meditation: Visualization

1. Sit in a comfortable position with your spine straight and close your eyes.
2. Take a few deep breaths and focus on your breath moving in and out of your body.
3. Once you've calmed your mind, begin to visualize a peaceful place. It can be anywhere you've been before or somewhere you've always wanted to go.
4. Visualize every detail of this place, from the colors to the sounds.
5. Spend at least 5 minutes in this visualization, then slowly open your eyes and take a few deep breaths.

Kriya Yoga is a powerful tool that can be used to improve your physical, mental, and emotional wellbeing. By combining asanas, mudras, mantras, and breathwork, you can create a practice that is tailored to your specific needs. Whether you're looking to boost your energy levels, relieve stress, or simply connect with your higher self, Kriya Yoga can help you achieve your goals. There you have it! Seven complete Kriya yoga routines that you can practice at home. Remember to listen to your body and do what feels comfortable for you.

Chapter 10: Your Daily Kriya Practice

When it comes to Kriya Yoga, consistency is key. In order for the techniques to have an effect on your life, you need to follow a proper routine. Now that you've learned about the various techniques involved in Kriya yoga, knowing where you should begin your practice can be quite confusing. This chapter will provide a detailed routine of various Kriya practices alongside Asanas, Pranayama, meditation, and Mudra techniques to guide you along the way. It's important that you're aware of how you should divide your Yoga time to get as much in your schedule as possible. Following this practice will be very simple, but the benefits will be extraordinary. This schedule is meant to be followed daily with a few variations.

Week 1

For the first week, you can choose from the following asana, meditation, and pranayama techniques for each day. It is suggested that you keep your daily practice to around 30 minutes, with 20 minutes for practicing asanas, 5 minutes for pranayama techniques, and the remaining 5 minutes for meditation. You can add 5 or 10 minutes of Mudras and Mantras if you want. Keep in mind that the techniques presented for the first week are the most basic and don't require any prior experience.

Asanas (20 min)

As you know by now, each asana has a unique benefit or specific purpose for which it is practiced. For the first week, you can choose from the following asanas. Before you start practicing these, do some basic stretching exercises. End the asana practice with a cooling-down pose, and remember to stay hydrated.

- **Goolf Ghoornan (Ankle Crank)**

Pose: Right knee bent and the foot placed on left thigh. The right hand supports the ankle, and the left hand holds the toes to rotate the foot.

Breathing: Inhale during the upward movement and exhale during the downward movement.

Awareness: On your breath and counting the rotations.

- **Ardha Titali Asana (Half Butterfly)**

Pose: One leg bent at the knee with the foot placed near the groin. Back bent with hands reaching the toes of the straight leg.

Breathing: Hold for 30 seconds while touching your toes. Exhale deeply.

Awareness: On your breathing and counting your breath.

- **Shroni Chakra (Hip Rotation)**

Pose: Right knee bent with the heel on the left thigh. The hip joint rotated in a circular motion.

Breathing: Inhale while carrying out the upward movement and exhale during the downward movement.

Awareness: On your breath, hip joints, rotations, any pressure or pain points, and waist position.

- **Utthanasana (Squat and Rise Pose)**

Pose: Knees bent sideways while standing, with buttocks lowered to assume a squatting position.

Breathing: Inhale while standing upright and exhale when lowering your buttocks and getting into position.

Awareness: On your breathing, the position of knees, and counting the squats.

- **Kawa Chalasana (Crow Walking)**

Pose: Feet kept apart in a squatting position with hands on the knees. One knee should be on the floor. With each step, the opposite knee should be on the floor.

Breathing: Normal, rhythmic breathing.

Awareness: On heartbeat, smoothness of steps, and muscles around the lower back, hips, and knees.

- **Saithaly Asana (Animal Relaxation Pose)**

Pose: Right knee bent with the foot resting near the inner left thigh. Left knee bent with the foot resting near right buttock. Torso turned to the right with head bent and resting on the right knee with arms stretched ahead.

Breathing: Inhale while getting into this position, and exhale when resting your head downwards.

Awareness: On your breathing, the muscles along the back, and counting the seconds.

- **Marjari Asana (Cat Stretch Pose)**

Pose: Resting on all fours with belly towards the ground, chin raised, and head tilted backward.

Breathing: Inhale and let your belly expand towards the floor. Exhale and suck in your stomach.

Awareness: On your spine, neck, and head movements.

Pranayama (5 min)

Pranayama is an important part of Kriya yoga practice, without which you will not be able to completely get into the relaxed state to practice meditation. While many people confuse pranayama with meditation, they are and should be treated differently. For the first week, pranayama should be done every day for five minutes. You can select any of the three techniques discussed below:

- **Sit in Sukhasana (easy pose)**

Pose: Legs crossed with hands resting on knees and palms open outwards.

Breathing: Right nostril closed using your right thumb. Inhale through the left nostril and hold for 5 seconds. Remove the thumb from the right nostril and exhale through it.

Awareness: On your breath and counting the seconds for each breath.

- **Yogic Breathing**

Pose: Cross-legged on the floor, or on a chair, with hands relaxed and spine upright.

Breathing: Inhale one-third of your lung capacity into the diaphragm; the next inhale should fill up your rib cage, and the third should expand your upper chest. In reverse order, exhale.

Awareness: On your breath as it moves into your lungs, on the movement of your muscles.

- **Samaveta Pranayama**

Pose: Any meditative asana in which you're comfortable and relaxed.

Breathing: Inhale through both nostrils and hold your breath for a second or two. Exhale slowly and hold your breath again for a second.

Awareness: On the rhythm of your inhales and exhales.

Meditation (5 min)

- **Naukasana (Boat Pose)**

Pose: Supine position with your feet stretched backward and arms behind your back.

Breathing: Inhale for 20 seconds and raise your body upwards. Hold for 4 seconds and exhale for another 20 seconds to bring your body back down.

Awareness: On your mind, breathing, and movement of muscles.

- **Hong Sau**

Pose: Spine straight, chest pushed outward at a 45-degree angle, with your chin outward.

Breathing: Inhale and exhale in a slow, rhythmic pattern.

Awareness: On your thoughts while chanting Hong and Sau. On your breath, as it enters through your nostrils and to your lungs. On the expansion and contraction of your chest.

Week 2

Once you've gotten used to practicing Kriya Yoga on a daily basis, you'll be able to handle more complex asanas, as well as advanced meditation techniques. Keep in mind that mastery of these techniques will not be achieved as soon as you start practicing but will only be possible through *consistent practice*. For the second week, you can choose from the following asana, meditation, and pranayama techniques for each day. For this week, you can increase the time of your meditative practice to 45 minutes, with 25 minutes dedicated to asana yoga, 10 minutes to meditation, and 10 minutes to pranayama. You can also add Mudras while performing meditation and pranayama techniques.

Asanas (25 min)

For the second week, you can choose from the following asanas. Before you start practicing these, do some basic stretching exercises. End the asana practice with a cooling-down pose, and remember to stay hydrated.

- **Chakki Chalanasana (churning the mill)**

Pose: Sitting position with legs wide apart, with both hands clasped and outstretched. The movement follows an imaginary circle with your clasped hands while moving your upper body.

Breathing: Inhale as you move your hands and body forward or to the right, and exhale as you're moving backward or to the left.

Awareness: On your breathing and muscles of your legs, groin, abs, and arms.

- **Gatyatmak Meru Vakrasana (dynamic spinal twist)**

Pose: With your legs apart and outstretched with arms reaching the toes of each foot. Make sure that your legs and arms don't bend.

Breathing: Inhale when your fingers touch your toes, and exhale as you get back into the initial position.

Awareness: On the torsional stretching of your spine and other muscle movements throughout your body.

- **Simha Kriya (lion's yawn)**

Pose: Kneeling position with both feet touching each other from the back. Hands placed on the floor while slightly leaning forward. Head tilted backward, and tongue folded backward, touching the back of the mouth.

Breathing: Inhale slowly through your nose in this position, and release your tongue at the end of the inhale. Exhale with your mouth and extend your tongue outwards while producing a steady vocal sound.

Awareness: On your breathing, the tension in your neck, and the sounds you make.

- **Shashankasana (moon pose)**

Pose: Buttocks resting on your feet with your hands on your thighs facing upwards. Arms raised above head and body bent to rest your head on your knees.

Breathing: Inhale when you stretch your arms and exhale when you bend to rest your head down. Retain your breath for 5 or 6 seconds before exhaling.

Awareness: On your breathing, stretching muscles, and counting rounds.

- **Sarpasana (snake pose)**

Pose: Lie down flat on your back, with legs straight and held together. Fingers interlocked and hands placed on buttocks. The chin is placed on the floor, and the body is raised as far back as possible.

Breathing: Inhale as you lift your body higher and exhale to let it back down.

Awareness: On your arms, legs, chest, and stiffness of muscles.

- **Bhujangasana (cobra pose)**

Pose: Belly facing the ground with legs stretched straight and toes holding your body upwards. Hands pressed lightly to the ground with your chest and head tilted backward.

Breathing: Inhale when you move your body upwards, and exhale to bring it down.

Awareness: On the tension of your muscles and your breathing.

Pranayama (10 min)

The pranayama techniques for the second week will be more advanced and will require some practice. Make sure you focus on your breathing more than your posture.

- **Plavini Pranayama**

Pose: Any meditative pose you feel comfortable in. Make sure that your spine should be straight and that your chest is pushed outwards.

Breathing: Breathe in through your mouth, letting the air fill your lungs. Close your mouth and hold your breath for a few seconds. Then, exhale deeply through the mouth while keeping it in a round shape.

Awareness: On your breathing and sense of tranquility that fills you with each inhale and exhale.

- **Nadi Shodhana**

Pose: Any meditation pose in which you have to sit upright.

Breathing: Inhale and exhale through the right nostril about 5 to 10 times while keeping the left one closed. Repeat this for the right nostril.

Awareness: On your breath as it moves through your nose and into your body.

Meditation (10 min)

- **Heartbeat Awareness**

Pose: Any meditation poses that you're comfortable in. Make sure that your spine is straight and your shoulders are back. Both of your hands should be placed on your heart.

Breathing: Deeply inhale and exhale.

Awareness: On the warmth of your hands, the rise and fall of your chest, and the beat of your heart as you inhale and exhale.

Following a guided schedule will ensure that you don't burn yourself out. While most of the initial yoga positions and techniques are easy, you'll need to practice the more complex ones to be able to master them. By practicing according to the provided schedule, you'll soon see a noticeable improvement.

Conclusion

Kriya yoga is a powerful spiritual practice that dates back over two thousand years. At its core, kriya yoga is all about self-realization – helping people uncover and fully embrace the divine truth of who they truly are. This involves a deep exploration of the mind, body, and spirit, working to clear out mental and emotional blockages to achieve greater awareness and inner peace. Through disciplined exercises, focused meditation, and positive affirmations, kriya yoga can help unlock one's potential for personal growth and enlightenment. It is also a challenging journey that requires focus, discipline, and dedication. If you are looking for a spiritual path that will lead you inward toward the heart of your being, then kriya yoga may be the perfect choice for you.

This easy-to-follow guide has introduced you to the basics of kriya yoga, from its history and key concepts to the essential techniques you need to get started on your journey of self-discovery. You have learned about the chakras, the subtle body, and how to use breathwork and meditation to connect with your higher self. You also explored the different asanas or kriya yoga poses that can help open up the energy channels in your body and promote deeper self-awareness. In addition, you have discovered how to combine all of these elements into a daily practice that will support your continued growth and transformation.

Kriya yoga is a comprehensive system of self-transformation that draws from many different elements and practices. Whether you are focusing on mantras, mudras, asanas, or pranayama, each step of kriya yoga is designed to help you move closer to your highest truth by clearing away negative energies and psychic blocks.

At the heart of kriya yoga is meditation, which is the primary practice through which you can achieve true inner stillness. By chanting mantras and focusing on positive thoughts or affirmations, you can quiet your mind and put yourself in a more receptive state that allows for greater insight and understanding. In addition to the benefits of meditation, kriya yoga also utilizes postures, breathing techniques, and hand motions to increase energy levels and promote balance on all levels of the self.

Whether you are new to kriya yoga or have been practicing it for years, there is always more to learn and explore in this rich tradition. With patience, dedication, and an open mind, each element of kriya yoga can lead you down the path toward enlightenment and ultimate wholeness.

When you first begin your kriya yoga practice, it is normal to feel somewhat overwhelmed by all the different poses, breathing techniques, and meditation practices involved. However, with time and patience, you'll start to build a firm foundation in the basics of this spiritual discipline. Once you have a solid understanding of how kriya yoga works and what it can do for you, it is time to take your practice to the next level. This may mean trying more challenging poses or focusing on incorporating certain elements like visualization into your meditation sessions.

Whatever your path may be, remember that every small step is an important one on your journey toward enlightenment. So, stay focused, remain disciplined, and keep pushing yourself to grow and evolve as a kriya yogi. Most importantly, always remember that this practice requires dedication – so stay committed and never give up on yourself!

Part 2: Turiya

The Ultimate Guide to Pure Consciousness, Hindu Philosophy, Samadhi, Shiva, and Shakti

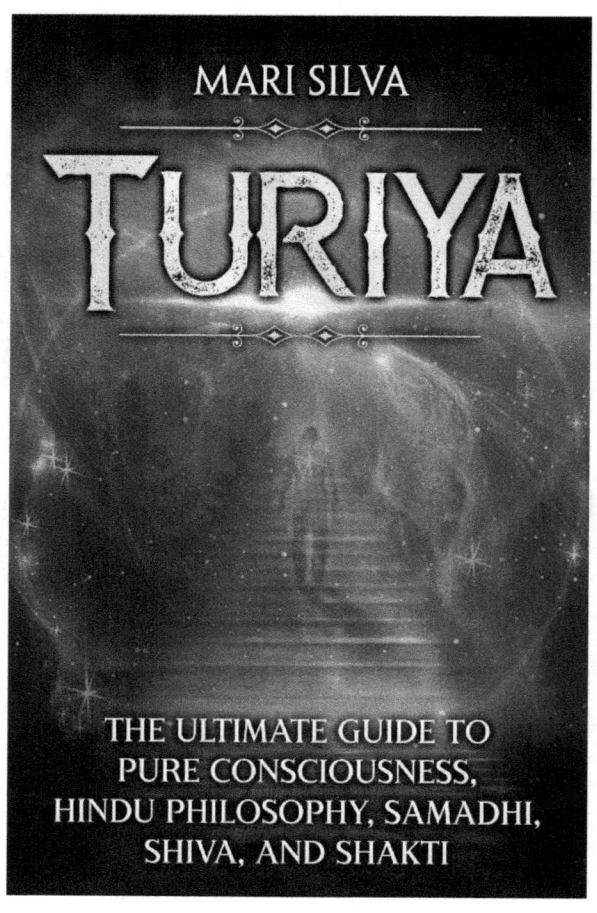

Introduction

Have you ever known what it's like to experience a state of pure consciousness? Complete bliss and oneness with the universe? This is what the Hindus call turiya, or *pure consciousness.*

Hindu philosophy is based on the belief that one supreme reality pervades and underlies all creation. This supreme reality is called Brahman, and it is the ultimate goal of all spiritual seekers. Brahman is often described as an infinite, omnipresent, and eternal ocean of consciousness. It is the source of all things and the goal of all things. Everything that exists is a part of Brahman, and everything is striving to return to Brahman.

This comprehensive guide will explore turiya, how it relates to Hindu philosophy, and how you can experience it through yoga and meditation. We'll also provide some practical tips and techniques you can use to pave the way to this ultimate state of awareness.

But before we dive in, there are some basics that we need to cover. We'll talk about Shiva and Shakti, the two essential aspects of Brahman. These two concepts are often misunderstood, so it's crucial to clearly understand them before we move on. Next, we'll discuss Samadhi, the goal of all yoga and meditation practices. Once we clearly understand these concepts, we'll explore turiya in greater depth.

Turiya is a state of pure consciousness that is beyond all duality. It is the fourth and final state of consciousness in the Hindu tradition. The first three states are waking, dreaming, and deep sleep. Turiya is beyond all of these states. It is a state of pure awareness that is limitless. Turiya is often described as a state of complete bliss. It's a state of being at one with the universe. In this state, there is no sense of separation between the observer and the observed. There is no sense of I or me. There is only pure awareness.

So how do we experience this state of pure consciousness? The information in this guide will show you. In this easy-to-understand guide, you'll also find yoga sequences, meditation techniques, and mantras that will help you experience turiya for yourself. You'll also learn about the daily steps you can take to bring yourself closer to this state of pure consciousness. We'll also dispel some common myths about turiya so that you can approach this topic with clarity and understanding.

By the end of this guide, you'll clearly understand what turiya is and how you can experience it for yourself. You'll also have a toolkit of practical techniques that you can use to pave the way to this ultimate state of awareness. So let's get started!

Chapter 1: What Is Turiya, or Pure Consciousness?

Have you ever found yourself wondering what consciousness is? You're not alone. The great philosophers and spiritual thinkers throughout history have all dedicated themselves to trying to understand the nature of consciousness. And while there are many different theories out there, one of the most intriguing comes from the Hindu tradition.

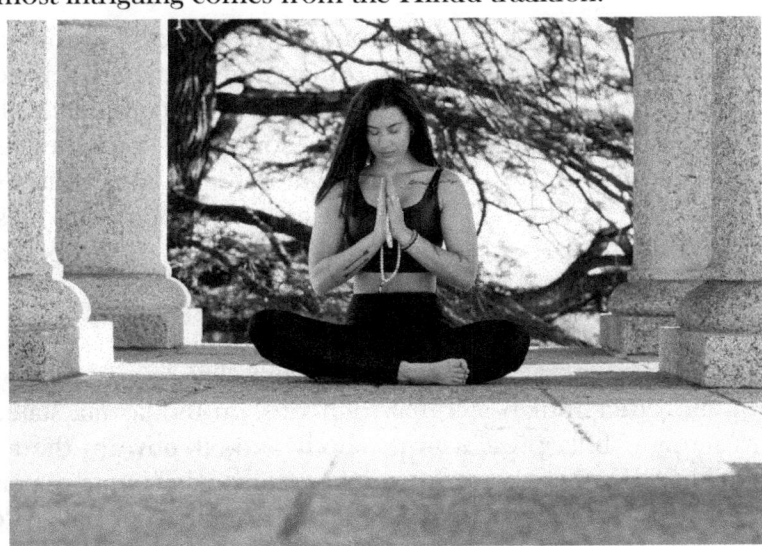

Turiya is described as the state of pure consciousness, the god state, or a great "cosmic silence."
https://www.pexels.com/photo/woman-in-black-tank-top-and-black-pants-sitting-on-concrete-floor-3820312/

In Hinduism, there is a concept known as turiya or pure consciousness. Its described as the state of pure consciousness, the god state, or a great "cosmic silence." To pave your way into thoroughly outlining what Turiya is, it might be best to first describe the four states of consciousness described by the Vedas and Upanishads: jagrata, svapna, susupti, and lastly, turiya.

This chapter will discuss the nature of consciousness according to Hinduism, focusing on the concept of turiya. We will explore how turiya is said to be different from the other three states of consciousness and how various Hindu traditions describe it. We will also look at accounts from gurus and experienced practitioners who have managed to access this state of pure consciousness. Finally, we will discuss how turiya has its stages.

The Four States of Consciousness

In the Hindu tradition, all humans regularly go through four distinct states of consciousness. The first of these is known as waking consciousness – when we are fully aware and awake. During this state, we experience life in full detail, interacting with our environment and taking in new information about the world around us. After a period of wakefulness comes dreaming, characterized by intense mental activity occurring while we sleep.

While our bodies rest, our minds continue to process information and generate ideas, creating vivid images and sensations. Next is deep sleep, or Susupti, which marks a phase where the mind rests completely. Finally, there is an even deeper state called Turiya – sometimes translated as 'pure awareness' – which involves an expanded state of consciousness that cannot be articulated entirely. Whether we are awake or asleep, these four states are an essential part of being human. Let's take a closer look at each one.

1. Jagrata: The Waking State

Jagrata, or "the waking state," is a concept that lies at the heart of Hinduism and other Indian spiritual traditions. In the jagrata state, one's awareness remains fully present in the body and attentive to the external world. Unlike in deep sleep or dreaming, a person in jagrata experiences complete lucidity, with all mental faculties functioning normally. Perhaps one of the key benefits of jagrata is that it gives rise to a clear understanding of one's own physical and mental limitations. By becoming more aware of how consciousness rises and subsides within us, we can develop mindfulness, which helps us to better navigate life's everyday challenges and experience greater peace and fulfillment. So whether you're seeking to deepen your spiritual practice or simply wish to live more mindfully, learning to stay in a state of jagrata may be just what you need.

2. Svapna: The Dreaming State

Svapna, or the dreaming state, has been another central concept in the two Hindu and Buddhist traditions for centuries. It refers to a state of mind in which one's consciousness separates from the physical body and travels freely through the spiritual realm. Some scholars claim this state can be induced through techniques such as yoga and meditation, while others believe that it will only occur spontaneously during sleep or intense spiritual practices. Regardless of its origins or mechanisms, many people view svapna as a powerful and transformative experience that offers insights into the nature of reality, self-knowledge, and enlightenment. Whether we fully understand it or not, svapna represents an essential part of our human experience, helping us to explore sides of ourselves that might otherwise remain hidden in our waking lives.

3. Susupti: The Deep Sleep State

Susupti is the Sanskrit word for a deep, dreamless sleep state. In this state, the body and mind fully relax and enter a state of complete rest. Though we may pass into susupti many times throughout the night as we sleep, it can also be experienced during moments of deep meditation or focus. Some scientists believe that the brain enters a strange kind of super-consciousness during these moments of susupti, allowing us to tap into our mental abilities in normally impossible ways. This may or may not be true, but there is no doubt that susupti holds great power and potential for anyone seeking greater levels of relaxation, inner peace, or insight. So why not take some time today to find your deep sleep state? With practice and patience, you will surely experience the incredible benefits of susupti for yourself.

4. Turiya: The State of Pure Consciousness

In many spiritual traditions, turiya is considered the ultimate state of consciousness. It's often described as a profound stillness that transcends all mental activity. In some ways, it can be thought of as a type of superconscious state where awareness is expanded to its fullest potential. Because it is beyond words or concepts, turiya can be difficult to fully grasp and understand. However, some have found that by cultivating certain techniques or practices, such as mindfulness or meditative techniques, one may eventually reach this extraordinary state of pure consciousness. Ultimately, turiya represents the ultimate goal of many aspiring seekers, beckoning us towards a deeper truth and harmony within ourselves.

Turiya beyond the Other Three States

Most traditions recognize that there is much more to consciousness than meets the eye. However, many traditions tend to focus on just one or two states at a time rather than exploring all aspects of consciousness in depth. While each state of consciousness is meaningful in its own right, it is also valuable to explore these states together, recognizing their interconnection and how they work together to create our overall experience. By doing so, we gain a deeper understanding of both ourselves and the world around us. And perhaps most importantly, we begin to realize that true enlightenment is not just about one particular state of mind; rather, it involves tapping into the full potential of human consciousness as a whole.

Ultimately, this limited perspective can hinder our spiritual development by limiting our perception of what lies beyond the other three states. To truly attain enlightenment - that is, to fully realize the potential of human consciousness - we must be willing and able to explore each dimension without attachment or aversion. Only then can we embark upon a truly transformative journey toward higher truth.

How Turiya Is Described in Various Hindu Traditions

Turiya, sometimes referred to as samadhi or ecstasy, is described very differently in various Hindu traditions. In Vedanta, turiya is described as a deep state of union with the divine, characterized by an overwhelming sense of timelessness and dissolution of individual identity. Maharishi Mahesh Yogi, one of the foremost yogic scholars of the 20th century, believed that turiya was attained through advanced meditation techniques and involved no cognitive awareness whatsoever. Conversely, Gaudapada and other members of the Shankara School describe turiya as more than just a spiritual state; they see it as a fundamental quality of reality itself. Regardless of the specific context in which it is discussed, one thing remains clear: turiya is profoundly transformative and has been revered throughout history by many different branches of Hinduism.

1. Vaishnavism

In the scriptures of Vaishnavism, turiya is a term often used to describe the ultimate state of spiritual awakening. This state represents a complete transcendence of all mental and sensory activity and is often equated with oneness with God. According to many Vaishnava texts, achieving this state requires intense dedication, deep begging practice, and constant devotion to the teachings of the sages. However, despite the challenges in attaining turiya, this state is believed to be attainable for anyone willing to put in the effort. With persistence and determination, even an ordinary person can achieve this greatly exalted spiritual state and experience true bliss. Ultimately, it can be said that turiya is one of the most precious gifts of Vaishnavism.

2. Shaivism

In the ancient Indian tradition of Shaivism, turiya is said to be the primordial energy and consciousness at the core of all existence. Often described as simultaneously transcendent and imminent, turiya is often conceived of as both formless and having a vast array of forms. With its immense powers, turiya is said to have created many aspects of reality, including universes, gods and goddesses, different levels of consciousness, and even sentient beings like humans and animals.

Not only is turiya seen as one of the most powerful forces in the universe, but it is also revered for its ability to awaken people's true potential. So, it's no surprise that many Shaivite practitioners strive to cultivate a close connection with this all-encompassing universal force. In essence, turiya can be thought of as the genesis of all that exists – both timeless and ever-changing, full of infinite wisdom yet bursting with endless creativity. Whether one connects with it through meditation, prayer, or other means, its power is undeniable, offering guidance and inspiration to anyone seeking it out.

3. Shaktism

In Shaktism, another tradition of Hinduism dedicated to the worship of the sacred feminine principle known as Shakti, turiya is often described as a divine force that permeates all aspects of the universe. This concept can be understood both spiritually and metaphysically. On the one hand, turiya is thought to manifest in sensory experience as an underlying presence that runs through all things, connecting them and infusing them with a sense of divinity. On the other hand, turiya also represents a transcendent state beyond the realm of duality and logic. In this sense, it points to a deeper reality that cannot be grasped by the mind or experienced with ordinary senses. Whether experienced on an individual or cosmic level, turiya is seen as essential for our understanding of life and the divine.

4. Smartism

In the tradition of Smartism, turiya is also often described as the highest spiritual state one can attain. This state represents a deep connection with one's true nature and opens up new realms of consciousness and understanding. To achieve this state, one must practice meditation and other forms of introspection daily. However, it is also essential to cultivate compassion for others, both human and non-human alike. By embracing turiya, we can find wisdom, peace, and freedom from suffering in our lives. Through this transformative process, we become more fully connected to the divine light within us all. While the path to reaching turiya may be long and challenging at times, it is worth every step along the way. Ultimately, turiya proves that our greatest power comes not from outside ourselves but from within ourselves.

5. The Vedas

In the Vedas, turiya is often described as an essential and sacred state of being. According to ancient wisdom traditions, turiya is the summit of human consciousness, and attaining this state can offer profound insights into the nature of reality. Furthermore, many spiritual masters believe that turiya represents the ultimate goal of all spiritual growth. This lofty state can be challenging, but those who devote themselves wholeheartedly to their inner development can unlock their full potential and achieve true enlightenment.

Ultimately, when we achieve control over our thoughts and feelings, turiya reveals itself as a deeply transformative experience that opens us up to new dimensions of being. With time, we gradually become more connected with the world around us and more in tune with our truest selves - our souls. Thus, turiya may be seen as one's journey toward realizing one's divine nature and becoming a reflection of universal truth and beauty.

6. The Upanishads

In the Upanishads, turiya is often described as a state of pure awareness and enlightenment. As one of four transcendent states of consciousness, turiya represents the ultimate goal of meditation and spiritual practice, where we become completely detached from the physical world and delve deeper into our true nature. Some scholars liken this state to reaching nirvana or achieving moksha, while others see it as an ongoing journey that encompasses all stages of life. Regardless of how we interpret this concept, there is no doubt that turiya represents one of the holiest and most profound concepts in Hinduism. Whether we seek to embody this ideal ourselves or simply integrate its teachings into our daily lives, the power and wisdom of turiya will continue to guide us on our path to greater understanding.

7. The Bhagavad Gita

According to the Bhagavad Gita, turiya is the ultimate state of consciousness. This state is said to be characterized by perfect stillness and awareness. It transcends all mental activity, allowing us to experience a deep sense of peace and serenity. Some have described turiya as a state of pure consciousness, where we are fully immersed in inner beauty and tranquility that extends beyond our perceived reality. Others view it as a merging with the divine or spiritual essence of all things, a transcendence that allows us to reconnect with our true nature and discover lasting joy and fulfillment. Regardless of how we choose to describe it, turiya has the power to awaken us to new levels of understanding and appreciation for ourselves, others, and the world around us. Whether we are seeking peace, clarity, or greater spiritual awareness, turiya holds the key.

8. The Yoga Sutras of Patanjali

Turiya is a mystical experience of being fully aware and present in the moment, beyond the limits of thought and language. According to the Yoga Sutra, this state can be reached by practicing regular meditation, focusing on clear perception and non-attachment to thoughts or objects. Turiya can also allow practitioners to experience higher states of empathy and compassion for others and to have a greater sense of connection with everything around them. Overall, turiya represents an opportunity for growth on both an individual and a spiritual level, and it is something that anyone interested in the deeper aspects of yoga should aspire to achieve.

9. Other Hindu Texts

Other Hindu texts also make mention of turiya, though it is often referred to by other names such as samadhi or nirvana. In the Mahabharata, for example, turiya is said to be in a state of complete detachment from the material world and complete absorption in the divine. The Ramayana illustrates Turiya as a state of absolute contentment, where an individual is free from worldly attachments and desires, and their soul has transcended the cycle of reincarnation. These texts illustrate the many different ways it can be understood, but they all point to the same ultimate goal: a state of complete and total liberation from the limitations of our physical reality.

Accounts of Gurus and Experienced Practitioners Who've Accessed Turiya

Accounts of gurus and experienced practitioners who have accessed the state known as turiya are some of the world's most fascinating and inspiring pieces of literature. These accounts tell of a state that transcends ordinary awareness and pushes one's consciousness to new heights. What is most remarkable about these accounts is not just what they describe but also how they describe it: with such vividness, precision, and detail that one can almost feel their experiences for themselves.

Many of these first-hand accounts focus on the sensation and experience of heightened awareness. Some describe a sense of unity with existence, filled with lightness, profound joy, boundlessness, and grace. Others speak of moments during which time seems to slow down or stop altogether and have an enhanced perception of reality. And still, others talk about experiencing higher levels of creativity, inspiration, and intuition beyond anything they had previously thought possible.

Whatever the specific nature or qualities they may have experienced while in this state, all these accounts paint a picture of turiya as being truly awe-inspiring and transformative. Whether people find themselves grappling with deep existential questions about life and death or simply marveling at the boundless beauty of the universe, what they learn while in this state invariably changes them forever. Through their words and experiences, we can begin to glimpse just how vast our inner worlds can be – if only we know where to look.

1. Ramana Maharshi

An influential Indian philosopher and mystical teacher, Ramana Maharshi, famously described his own experience of accessing the turiya in one of his writings. In his account, he explains that after experiencing a profound sense of inner stillness, he was suddenly awakened to the fact that he existed on a much more fundamental level than he had previously believed. At the core of his being, all thoughts, emotions, and desires seemed to dissolve into nothingness. Through this transformative encounter with the turiya, Ramana came to fully understand the underlying unity between himself and all beings in the universe. Whether or not we have had similar experiences ourselves, his story offers us an intriguing glimpse into this elusive dimension of consciousness.

2. Nisargadatta Maharaj

Nisargadatta Maharaj was one of the most influential spiritual teachers of his time, known for his profound insights into the nature of consciousness and reality. Although Maharaj was highly respected by his followers, he attributed his globally renowned awakening to a process that was quite straightforward. According to his account, it all began when he had an epiphany one evening while sitting under the stars. He suddenly realized that he was no different from those twinkling lights in the sky since everything – even himself – is ultimately an expression of the same underlying consciousness. Knowing this truth at an intuitive level allowed him to access something far greater than ourselves, which he referred to as turiya – or pure awareness without thoughts or feelings. Although many were initially skeptical of Maharaj's claims, over time, more and more people came to recognize the validity and wisdom behind his teachings on self-realization.

3. Swami Vivekananda

For centuries, philosophers and spiritual teachers have sought to explain the mysteries of the human mind. While some believed that the ultimate state of being could only be reached through meditation or intense intellectual study, Swami Vivekananda believed that it was possible to achieve this advanced state by engaging in certain physical practices. The fourth state of consciousness, turiya, can be accessed by anyone who learns to still their mind and body. By following his unique instructions for physically connecting with one's inner being, Vivekananda claimed that anyone could unlock their full potential and access turiya.

Through experiencing this exalted state for themselves, individuals would gain unparalleled insights into the nature of reality itself. In this rapidly evolving world, we are constantly challenged to push ourselves impossibly further and reach new heights. Many people today credit the teachings of Swami Vivekananda with providing them with the tools they need to navigate this ever-changing landscape, unlocking their true potential and discovering direct knowledge of reality. Through his transformative wisdom, Vivekananda offers us a unique perspective on the human experience, encouraging us to find meaning within ourselves instead of chasing after external validation.

The Stages of Turiya

Throughout the ancient texts of yoga and Hindu philosophy, we find references to a distinct state of consciousness known as turiya. The word turiya is derived from two Sanskrit words meaning "fourth" and "state." This refers to the fact that this state is the fourth or highest level of consciousness. There are several specific stages or phases associated with Turiya avastha, including Sahaja avastha (the natural or innate state), kevala avastha (the absolute state), and turyatita avastha (the fifth, or highest, phase). While it is clear that each stage represents a deepening awareness and a further opening of our consciousness to higher levels of reality, there is still much unknown about this mysterious, transformative state. Nonetheless, anyone who wishes to explore their potential for spiritual awakening would do well to begin by looking within themselves for the true experience of turiya.

Sahaja Avastha: The Natural State

In the sahaja avastha or natural state, we access our highest level of consciousness without any effort or training. This is the state of true self-realization, in which we spontaneously awaken to our divine nature and experience a deep sense of peace and bliss. This state is also called "the constant state" because it is our natural default setting. We all have the potential to live in this state permanently, but we often get caught up in the noise and clutter of our minds, which obscures our true nature and prevents us from accessing the peace and bliss that is possible.

Kevala Avastha: The Absolute State

The kevala avastha, or absolute state, is one of pure consciousness, free from all conceptual limitations. In this state, we are no longer identified with our thoughts, emotions, or physical bodies. We are simply aware of being and experience a deep sense of peace and unity with all creation. This state is also known as "the witness state" because we observe the play of creation without getting caught up in it. We remain centered in our true nature, regardless of what is happening around us.

Turyatita Avastha: The Highest State

The turyatita avastha, or highest state, is a state of complete transcendence. This is when we are no longer aware of even our existence. We are one with the absolute and experience a deep sense of peace and bliss. This state is also known as "the state beyond turiya" because it is beyond all conceptual limitations. In this state, we are no longer bound by time or space, and we experience a deep sense of unity with all of creation.

Turiya, or "the fourth state," is a concept that is deeply embedded in many Hindu traditions. While different denominations and lineages describe this state of consciousness differently, they all agree that it is the highest possible state of being. Some believe Turiya is a transcendent reality beyond time and space, while others view it as an underlying state of awareness that permeates waking and dreaming experiences.

Experts who have accessed this state of pure consciousness describe it as a state of complete peace and bliss. In this state, we are no longer identified with our thoughts, emotions, or physical bodies. We are simply aware of being and experience a deep sense of unity with all creation. While turiya is the highest state of consciousness, it is also the most difficult to access. It requires a great deal of spiritual training and practice to achieve.

There are several stages or phases associated with turiya avastha, including sahaja avastha (the natural or innate state), kevala avastha (the absolute state), and turyatita avastha (the highest state). Each stage represents a deepening of awareness and a further opening of our consciousness to higher levels of reality. Learning about and experiencing these stages can help us to understand our potential for spiritual growth and awakening.

While the concept of turiya may be difficult to grasp, we all have the potential to experience this state of pure consciousness. It is our birthright. With practice and dedication, we can all access the peace and bliss of turiya avastha.

Chapter 2: Hindu Philosophy Basics

Hindu philosophy is a complex and multifaceted subject encompassing several different schools of thought and beliefs. Depending on one's perspective, Hindu philosophy can be seen as an endless tapestry of ideas and concepts or as a deeply interconnected system of traditional wisdom. Some common themes central to much Hindu thought include the importance of karma, the goal of liberation from worldly suffering, the belief in reincarnation, and the idea that all living things are intrinsically connected through a universal consciousness.

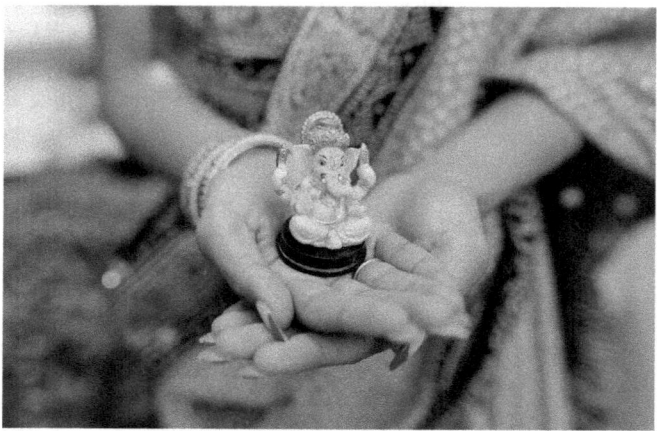

Hindu philosophy is a complex and multifaceted subject, encompassing several different schools of thought and beliefs.
https://www.pexels.com/photo/person-holding-an-elephant-figurine-7685576/

Regardless of one's particular interpretation of these concepts, they form the core of the rich tradition that is Hindu philosophy. Ultimately, it is up to each person to take what resonates with them from this fascinating topic and incorporate it into their understanding of the world. In this chapter, we will explore some key ideas and schools of thought within Hindu philosophy to better understand this complex and ancient system of thought.

The Nature of the Soul

According to the Hindu philosophy of Advaita Vedanta, the soul is a fundamental, unchanging part of all living beings. This idea is grounded in the belief that all matter is interconnected, with each individual being deeply connected to the world around them. In this view, our souls are not separate from nature but rather an integral part of it. In this view, our souls are not separate from nature but rather an integral part of it. This concept is often called "the unity of all things." Given these central tenets of Hindu thought, it is clear that one's soul is seen as something intimately connected to and reflective of the natural world as a whole. At its essence, the nature of the soul, as conceived by Hindu philosophy, is defined by harmony and unity with all life.

Consciousness

Consciousness is one of the fundamental principles central to the Hindu philosophy of Vedanta. According to this philosophy, consciousness is not only what allows us to experience the world around us, but it is also what gives rise to all aspects of our reality and existence. In other words, consciousness is considered the root of our outer and inner worlds and guides our thoughts, feelings, and actions.

Hindu philosophers believe that consciousness can take on many different forms or layers. For example, there is a deep sentient level of consciousness that permeates every aspect of reality, and there are also minute vessels or particles that carry this universal consciousness throughout the universe. While we may tend to think about consciousness in terms of human minds or individual awareness, these Hindus believe that it envelops all things in both an infinite and finite sense. Therefore, according to Hinduism, understanding this concept is key for anyone wishing to fully grasp the nature of reality.

The World

According to Hindu philosophy, the world is a veil of illusion that obscures our true selves from view. From this perspective, everything in the universe – from our most cherished relationships to the foods we eat and our possessions – is merely a temporary manifestation of an underlying eternal reality. This idea plays out in many different ways in Hindu thought, but perhaps one of its most powerful concepts is the emphasis on harmonious coexistence between humans and nature. Indeed, Hindu scriptures view the earth as a living being filled with divine energy, or prana, and argue that all people must respect and nurture this energy if they want to sustain life on this planet.

Whether we are looking at ancient Hindu teachings or modern-day practices such as organic farming and renewable energy, it's clear this worldview has profoundly impacted how Hindus view their relationship with the natural world. At its heart, then, Hindu philosophy is not just a system of spiritual beliefs; it is also an environmental ethic that calls us all to cherish and protect our beautiful planet.

Prana

Prana, or life energy, is an essential concept in Hindu philosophy. According to ancient teachings, prana is one of the primary elements of the universe, providing the vital force that allows all living things to grow and thrive. In humans, prana flows through the breath and circulates throughout the body via a complex network of energy channels called nadis. Followers believe that regulating the flow of prana through these channels can have far-reaching benefits for both physical and mental health.

Practicing breathing and meditation techniques is believed to increase the amount of prana in their bodies and improve their overall sense of well-being. So, while prana may be a difficult concept to fully understand from an academic perspective, it is a key part of traditional Hindu thought and a crucial part of spiritual practice.

The Chakras

According to ancient Hindu philosophy, seven major energy centers are called chakras. Located throughout the body, these chakras represent different aspects of our being, from physical and mental makeup to spiritual outlook. Each chakra holds different colored energy that radiates outward through channels known as nadis. Through practices like yoga and meditation, we can learn to harness this energy to achieve harmony and balance in our lives. Whether you seek greater strength and vitality or a deeper sense of connection with the universe, paying close attention to the state of your chakras may help you on your journey. Here's a list of the seven chakras and their associated meanings:

The Root Chakra (Muladhara): Located at the base of the spine, this chakra is associated with our most basic survival instincts. It governs our sense of safety and security and helps us feel grounded and connected to the earth.

The Sacral Chakra (Swadhisthana): This chakra is located just below the navel and is associated with the element of water. It governs our emotions and is responsible for our creativity and sexual energy.

The Solar Plexus Chakra (Manipura): This chakra is located in the solar plexus area, just below the sternum. It is associated with the element of fire and governs our sense of personal power and self-esteem.

The Heart Chakra (Anahata): The Anahata chakra, which roughly translates to "unhurt" or "undamaged," is located in the center of the chest. It's often symbolized by the air element due to its representation of intellectual capacity and spirituality. It governs our ability to love and be loved and is responsible for our sense of compassion and empathy.

The Throat Chakra (Vishuddha): This chakra is located in the throat area and is associated with the element of ether. It governs our ability to communicate and is responsible for our sense of truthfulness and integrity.

The Third Eye Chakra (Ajna): This chakra is located between the eyebrows and is associated with the element of mind. It governs our ability to see clearly and is responsible for our intuition and imagination.

The Crown Chakra (Sahasrara): The crown chakra, located at the top of the head, is associated with spiritual energy. It governs our connection to the divine and is responsible for our sense of enlightenment and spiritual wisdom.

By working with the chakras, we can learn to cultivate greater health, happiness, and harmony in our lives. Through practices like yoga and meditation, we can understand the role these energy centers play in our overall well-being.

Atman

Atman, or "self," is a fundamental concept in Hindu philosophy that refers to the essence of an individual. In Hindu belief, Atman unites all living beings, and it exists regardless of one's outward appearance or circumstances. While each person's Atman may be unique and individual, it is also interconnected with the larger universe. According to Hindu teachings, the ultimate goal in life is to realize our true nature as Atman and unite with the divine consciousness of Brahman. Through meditation, devotion, and wisdom, we can tap into the limitless potential of our souls and find lasting happiness and fulfillment. Whether we fully understand its meaning or not, Atman remains a central concept in Hindu thought that serves as a source of inspiration for us all.

Brahman

The concept of Brahman is at the heart of Hindu philosophy and spirituality. This is a highly abstract notion, so it can be difficult to fully understand its significance and meaning. However, at its core, Brahman is understood to represent the soul or essence of the universe. It is seen as the source of all creation and is often described as a vast, unlimited creative energy. By cultivating an awareness of this energy within ourselves, we can better understand our place in the cosmos and come closer to attaining spiritual enlightenment. So, for many Hindus, Brahman represents an ultimate truth about existence and an essential guiding principle for living a meaningful life.

Karma

According to the ancient Hindu philosophy of karma, all our actions are governed by a universal cycle of cause and effect. Whether we are aware of it or not, every time we make a decision, take action, or speak a word, we contribute to this worldview and, in turn, shape our destiny. While some may view karma simply as a system of rewards and punishments for our actions, others see it as a tool for spiritual growth and self-discovery. Regardless of how one interprets this complex philosophy, the principle of karma is deeply meaningful for many Hindus and continues to influence their lives and culture today. Essentially, it is a reminder that our choices have far-reaching consequences for us and those around us. And ultimately, our interactions with the world shape who we become.

Moksha

Moksha, or spiritual liberation, is another tenet central to Hindu philosophy. According to this ancient belief system, achieving moksha requires detachment from worldly things and reaching a state of union with Brahman, the divine essence that permeates all creation. This process can involve various stages or levels of enlightenment, including jnana yoga, the path of wisdom; karma yoga, the path of action; and bhakti yoga, the path of devotion. Ultimately, however, moksha is less about a specific set of practices or beliefs and more about a state of absolute freedom and transcendence from suffering. So whether you are looking for inner peace, emotional equanimity, or spiritual awakening, the core idea behind Moksha offers an excellent guiding principle on your journey towards higher consciousness.

Samsara

In Hindu philosophy, samsara is often described as a cyclical pattern of birth, death, and rebirth. According to this widely-accepted worldview, our current lives are just one stage in a constantly moving cycle of existence. To free ourselves from this endless spiral and achieve true liberation, we must first understand the nature of samsara and what it takes to escape it. This can be accomplished through diligent spiritual practice and devotion to the divine truth. Ultimately, Hindu teachings hold that samsara represents an illusion that can be overcome with wisdom and spiritual insight. Only by embracing this liberating truth can we transcend the endless cycle once and for all

Yoga

Yoga is a practice that has been integral to Hindu philosophy for thousands of years. For ancient Hindus, yoga was not simply a series of exercises and meditations aimed at achieving physical or mental breakthroughs. Rather, it was seen as a spiritual path with transformative powers, guiding practitioners toward developing closer connections with the natural world and their fellow humans.

Today, modern yoga continues to be influenced by these timeless teachings, focusing on quieter movements and deeper breathing as ways to tap into hidden parts of the self. Whether you are hoping to achieve physical flexibility or are simply searching for a way to enhance your meditation routine, yoga offers abundant benefits to help you reconnect with your innermost being. So what are you waiting for? Step onto your mat and start exploring this ancient spiritual practice today!

The Three Gunas

According to ancient Hindu philosophy, three basic "gunas," or personality characteristics, govern all living creatures. The first is sattva, meaning "purity" or "goodness." Individuals with a predominantly sattvic nature tend to be calm, centered, and compassionate. The second is rajas, which means "passion" or "aggression." Those with a strong rajasic quality are dynamic and driven, always looking for new challenges to conquer.

Finally, there is tamas, which can be thought of as the slothful guna. Individuals who display this quality tend to be lazy and resistant to change; they also often struggle with depression and despair. While no one individual will embody only one of these gunas, most people do have an innate leaning towards one or more of these personalities. Understanding the different gunas can help us better understand ourselves and others around us.

The Four Noble Truths

The Four Noble Truths are an essential concept in Hindu philosophy. According to these Truths, life is characterized by suffering and dissatisfaction, and the root cause of this dissatisfaction is desire. To achieve liberation from this struggle, we must first recognize the true nature of our desires and understand that these wants will never fully satisfy us. Once we have achieved this understanding, we can move on to the second Noble Truth: that the way to eliminate our desires is through a process of self-discipline and meditation. Finally, through practice and discipline, we can begin to overcome negative emotions such as anger or jealousy, ultimately freeing ourselves from suffering and reaching a state of true enlightenment.

The third and fourth Noble Truths offer a roadmap for reaching this goal, offering practical advice to help us on our journey toward liberation. These Truths are a pivotal part of Hindu philosophy and offer valuable insights into the human condition. Whether familiar with Hindu philosophy or not, these Noble Truths provide a crucial framework for living a better life. If you struggle to find satisfaction in your life, consider exploring the Four Noble Truths further. They just might hold the key to true happiness.

The Eightfold Path

An Eightfold Path is another powerful tool for spiritual growth and enlightenment. This path consists of eight different practices or attitudes, each of which is essential in achieving higher levels of consciousness. These include the right view, right aspiration, right speech, right conduct, right livelihood, right effort, right mindfulness, and finally, right concentration. By committing to these aspects of the Eightfold Path, one can cultivate greater wisdom and awareness both in your own life and in your interactions with others. One can find true happiness and fulfillment by embracing the holistic approach offered by this path and striving for continued self-development and transformation.

The Interconnection of All Things

In Hindu philosophy, everything in the universe is considered to be interconnected at a fundamental level. This idea is reflected in the concept of karma, which holds that every action has consequences that play out on both a personal and cosmic scale. The interconnectedness of all things also extends to our physical environment, as nearly every living thing on Earth relies on natural resources that must be continually replenished by birth, growth, and death cycles.

In this way, humanity is responsible for caring for and safeguarding the natural world around us for the sake of our karmic well-being and for generations to come. So whether you're a devoted yogi or simply someone who appreciates the wonders of nature, it's clear that grounding yourself in an understanding of interconnection can help you appreciate your place in the vast web of life. After all, what we do now really does matter.

Dharma

Dharma, or dharma according to the Hindu philosophy, is another central element in the religion and culture of India. While it has several different meanings depending on the context, Dharma is generally understood as a set of moral principles or duties that guide individuals and society. For example, one of the most basic concepts of dharma is Rita, or the right way to live according to the laws of nature. This includes performing honest work, caring for those in need, and living in harmony with all living things. Dharma also shapes social interactions among individuals, which includes respecting elders and holding family members accountable for their actions. At a more metaphysical level, dharma is also understood as the underlying principle of cosmic order and justice. In this sense, it represents the universe's natural balance and energy flow.

Satya

In Hindu philosophy, Satya is one of the cardinal virtues. This concept, translated as truthfulness or sincerity, holds that each person's words and actions should be intrinsically good and reflect their innermost beliefs. Satya embodies an overarching goal for the religious devotee to embody goodness in everything they do, from how they treat others to how they conduct themselves in their day-to-day life.

Practicing Satya is a personal journey needing constant reflection and awareness. It requires us to be mindful in our interactions with others and introspective about our motives and goals. Though it may be difficult at times to maintain this level of integrity and honesty in our daily lives, those who can pursue this virtuous path will undoubtedly be rewarded for their efforts both on a spiritual plane and in their relationships with others. Ultimately, by striving to live by the tenets of Satya, we can truly become the authentic people we were always meant to be.

Artha

Artha refers to the pursuit of social and economic prosperity. This concept includes any activities that help us achieve wealth, power, and prestige. While many people view artha as a wholly materialistic pursuit, this perspective ignores the fact that it is intimately intertwined with an individual's mental, spiritual, and emotional well-being. After all, having money and status can help to improve our quality of life by providing security and allowing us to support our family. Artha also encourages us to be driven and goal-oriented, which helps us achieve great things in life and furthers society as a whole. In short, artha is an essential part of the human experience that should be embraced rather than shunned.

Dwaita, Adwaita, and Vishishtadwaita

Dwaita, Adwaita, and Vishishtadvaita are three major schools of thought within Hindu philosophy. Dwaita, which can be translated as dualism, posits that there is a fundamental distinction between the individual soul (atman) and the universal soul (Brahman). This view holds that the individual soul is an eternal and immortal entity, while the universal soul is an impersonal force that governs the universe. For followers of Dwaita, atman and brahman are completely separate entities, while those who follow Adwaita believe that they are ultimately identical. In contrast, adherents to Vishishtadvaita believe that atman and brahman possess some qualities in common but are by no means the same.

Though Dwaita is generally seen as the oldest school of thought within Hindu philosophy, each approach has its own rich history and traditions that continue to influence new generations of thinkers today. Perhaps most importantly, these schools all seek to answer a central question: how can we achieve moksha or liberation from suffering? While there is certainly considerable debate around this question, they all agree that spiritual knowledge is key to attaining moksha. Through their interpretations of atman and brahman, as well as through their teachings on spirituality and other aspects of life, these three schools continue to shape our understanding of Hinduism and its central beliefs.

Hindu philosophy is a complex and varied field that encompasses a wide range of beliefs and practices. At its core, however, Hinduism focuses on the individual's journey to spiritual enlightenment. This goal is achieved through various means, including the pursuit of knowledge, self-reflection, and virtuous living. Though the path to moksha, or liberation from suffering, is often difficult, those who follow it can achieve great rewards both on a spiritual and a material level. By understanding the basics of Hindu philosophy, we can gain a greater appreciation for this rich tradition and its impact on the world.

Chapter 3: Shakti and Shiva, a Divine Union

Shakti and Shiva are two well-known Hindu deities representing specific energies: Shakti (the feminine divine) and Shiva (the masculine divine.). Though often thought of and worshipped as two separate entities, they are two halves of the same whole, and their union is essential to create balance in the universe. In Hinduism, the balance of masculine and feminine energy is considered essential for both individual well-being and the health of the cosmos.

In this chapter, we will first explore Shakti – her symbolism, portrayal, and the significance of her energy. We will then do the same for Shiva before discussing the significance of their union and how it relates to our own lives. By understanding the nature of Shakti and Shiva, we can understand life's deeper mysteries.

Shakti - The Feminine Divine

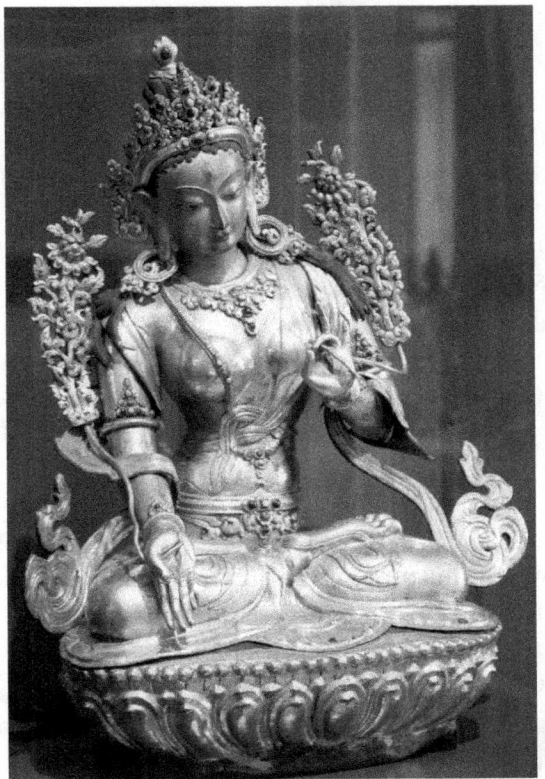

Shakti - The Feminine Divine.
https://pixabay.com/es/photos/museo-rietberg-arte-de-asia-shiva-66868/

Shakti is a multifaceted concept representing the divine feminine in both Hindu and Buddhist traditions. In Hinduism, Shakti is seen as the feminine counterpart to Shiva, the overarching masculine principle of the universe. Together, these two deities embody all aspects of creation and destruction in the cosmos. However, Shakti also exists independently, distinct from Shiva as an individual goddess in her own right. Shakti is the divine feminine energy of the universe, revered in many religious and spiritual traditions worldwide.

In Buddhism, Shakti represents latent or potential energy that can be activated through spiritual practice. Whether viewed as a representation of divine power or an internal force within ourselves, Shakti is a powerful symbol of female strength and resilience. Indeed, it is no accident that women often call upon this beloved archetype when times are tough, and they need help carrying on. Whether you look to her for support or guidance, there is no doubt that Shakti embodies all that is powerful about femininity.

Symbolism

At its core, Shakti represents the creative power and transformative energy flowing through all things. She can be seen as a representation of the cycles of nature - birth, growth, decay, death, and regeneration - as well as the grounding forces such as intuition and emotion. Her sacred symbols can be found in everything from temple art to everyday household items women use.

Shakti's symbol is the yoni, a Sanskrit word meaning "womb" or "origin." The yoni is often depicted as a triangular shape, representing the creative power of the universe. It is through the yoni that all things are born, and it is also through the yoni that they will eventually return. The yoni symbolizes Shakti's creative energy, reminding us that all things are connected.

By acknowledging and honoring Shakti's presence in our lives, we can draw on her power to nurture and protect us, guiding us along our path of growth and transformation. After all, without Shakti at the helm, there would be no life or change, or growth at all. She remains one of the most significant symbols of spirituality we know today.

Portrayal

Throughout history, the powerful feminine divine has been portrayed in many different ways. In Buddhism, Shakti is sometimes portrayed as a wrathful goddess, such as the popular deity Tara. Tara is often shown with multiple arms, each holding a different weapon or tool. This represents her ability to protect and defend those who call upon her. Other times, Shakti is portrayed as a peaceful goddess, such as Kuan Yin, the popular Chinese deity of compassion. Perhaps one of the most famous depictions of this goddess is in the Devi Mahatmya, a Sanskrit text that describes her as a fierce warrior who battles demons to protect humanity.

Similarly, in Hindu art and sculpture, she is shown wielding weapons such as swords and tridents, symbolizing her strength and courage. They are a strong reminder of the power and beauty of Shakti. Through them, we are reminded that women have played an integral role in shaping our world for the better and that we should continue celebrating their strength and wisdom for generations to come. In Hindu art, Shakti is often shown holding a trident, symbolizing her power over the three aspects of reality -

mind, body, and spirit.

Shakti is also often shown riding a lion, signifying her role as the supreme ruler of the animal kingdom. She is also pictured holding a lotus flower in some depictions, symbolizing her connection to the natural world. The lotus symbolizes purity and rebirth, reminding us that Shakti is always with us, even in the darkest times.

Manifestation

The energy of Shakti has many different manifestations within and around us, taking on different forms depending on where we are and what we are doing. For example, Shakti can appear as a kind, motherly figure during times of tranquility and peace, offering comfort and support to those who need it. At other times, Shakti may manifest as a fierce warrior, defending us against all odds and helping us to overcome any challenges we face.

Regardless of how she chooses to present herself, Shakti is always there within us or around us, ready at any moment to help guide us along our paths in life. Whether we realize it or not, this powerful energy is always at work, manifesting wisdom and compassion in subtle and overt ways. When we pay attention to this divine feminine energy within and around us, we open ourselves up to all of the gifts she offers.

Power and Significance

Regardless of its particular manifestation, Shakti epitomizes all that is feminine and powerful. With her boundless energy, she shapes and sustains the world, instilling in all living beings the strength and vitality necessary for survival. In this sense, she plays a vital role in both the cosmos and our lives, reminding us of our innate power and significance amidst our intense struggles.

In times of hardship, Shakti gives us the courage to persevere and the will to overcome obstacles in our path. Her energy also fills us with hope, reminding us that no matter how dark or difficult our journey may be, we always have the potential to rise and blossom into something beautiful. Shakti is the force that drives us to live and love fully; through her power, we create and manifest our reality. Shakti serves as an external reminder of our inner strength and a constant source of guidance and comfort on our path through life.

Associate Deities

Shakti is the name given to various Hindu goddesses representing different aspects of femininity and the divine feminine. While there are hundreds of different Shaktis, some of the most revered include Durga, Kali, and Parvati. Each of these goddesses embodies a specific set of qualities, ranging from unrelenting force to soft, maternal love. Together, they form a complex web of associations with Shakti as both protector and nurturer. Whether you seek guidance or solace in your journey, there is sure to be an associated deity of Shakti that can provide the support you need. So if you are searching for strength in hard times or compassion in difficult situations, look no further than the many splendors of Shakti's divine feminine power.

Shiva - The Masculine Divine

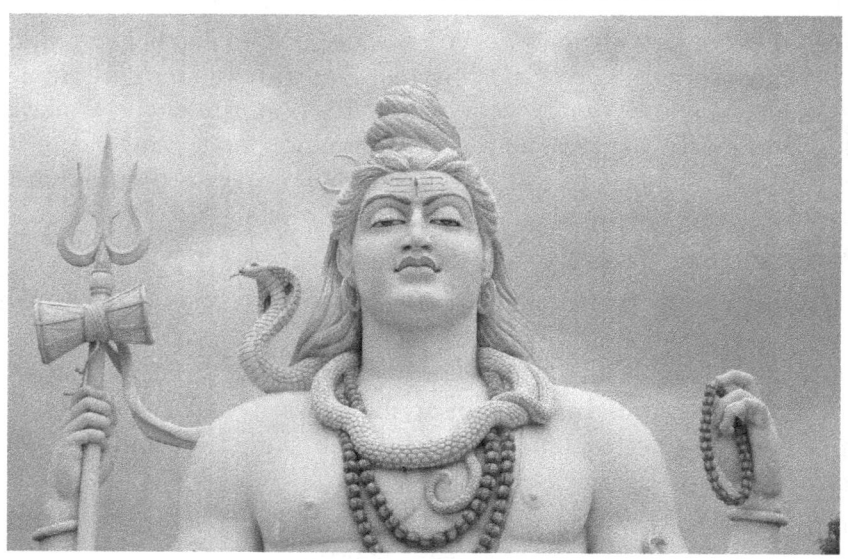

Shiva - The Masculine Divine.
https://www.pexels.com/photo/statue-of-shiva-5935661/

Often portrayed as both the divine destroyer and the divine creator, Shiva is one of the most widely worshipped deities in Hinduism. Many consider him to be the embodiment of masculinity, embodying qualities such as power, strength, and virility. His many forms include that of a fearsome warrior, a benevolent king, and even a playful child. By honoring his power and complexity, devotees seek to connect with their inner masculine energy and cultivate it in beneficial ways. Whether through meditation, prayer, or spiritual devotion, many Hindus view Shiva as an important figure to help guide them on their journey toward spiritual growth.

Symbolism

The Hindu deity Shiva is often depicted as the symbol of the masculine divine, a fierce and powerful god who wields both a trident and fire, and he is closely associated with destruction, change, and transformation. Shiva's symbolism draws on many different elements, from his various names invoking various aspects of nature to the myths surrounding him that connect him with creation and rebirth.

Perhaps most significantly, though, Shiva's archetypal masculinity links him to primal forces and energies that are central to the universe's functioning. Through his portrayal in mythology and art, Shiva represents one of the fundamental building blocks of existence. He also reminds us that all things must be allowed to change so continued growth and renewal can occur. In this sense, Shiva truly embodies the symbolic nature of the masculine divine.

Purification

In many ancient traditions, purification holds a special significance. In Hinduism, the power of purification is associated with Shiva, the supreme god and source of all creation. Shiva embodies the qualities of strength, potency, and authority that are often associated with male energy. Purification also symbolizes cleansing and rejuvenation, two concepts central to many spiritual practices.

With this in mind, it becomes clear why Shiva has long been seen as a significant figure in helping seekers and meditators understand their true nature and purpose in life. Through intense meditation on all things pure and sacred, one can come closer to truly embodying the essence of Shiva, opening oneself up to a lifetime of spiritual insight and growth. Thus, when it comes to purifying ourselves physically and spiritually, few figures carry as much weight as the mighty deity known as Shiva.

Transformation

As one of the most prominent deities in the Hindu tradition, Lord Shiva is also known for his transformative powers. Perhaps the best-known example of this is in his relationship with his consort Parvati. The masculine divine had been begging for rebirth as a child to experience unconditional love and devotion once again, and when Parvati offered to be his mother, he finally relented.

With her love and support, Shiva fully embraced his feminine side, overcoming all of his negative qualities and transcending into something purer and more beautiful than ever. Through this process, Shiva came to embody masculine and feminine principles at once, proving himself an example of perfect harmony and unity. In essence, through transforming ourselves, we can truly come in touch with our true nature - that of the sacred force of creation embodied within us all.

Power and Significance

In many ancient cultures and religions, power and significance have long been associated with the divine masculine. Among these religions is the Hindu tradition of Shaivism, which centers around the figure of Shiva as a symbol of masculine potency. For those who follow Shaivism, this powerful god symbolizes strength, power, virtue, and fertility.

Shiva is often depicted as a wild god, dancing wildly on mountaintops with serpents draped around his body. It is this raw energy that gives Shiva a powerful significance in the eyes of his followers. However, this sense of absolute power can be balanced out by his other characteristic attributes - such as compassion for his devotees and wisdom in his teachings. In this way, Shaivism offers an ideal representation of how the divine masculine can be a source both of immense power and deep wisdom. With this unique duality at its core, it's no surprise that this ancient religion continues to inspire believers today.

Energy Manifestation

Shiva, the Hindu god of destruction, is often associated with energy manifestation. This is because he brings about change through both destruction and renewal. Through his cosmic dance, for example, Shiva destroyed the world to create it anew. In addition, he is also linked with the cycles of life and death that are an essential part of any material existence. At the same time, Shiva embodies the masculine divine, representing the universal force that sustains all things. These two sides of Shiva's nature make him a powerful symbol of transformation and growth.

Whether by destroying what no longer serves us or creating new opportunities for change in our lives, we can all learn to harness some of this energy and manifest power within us. After all, change is an inevitable and integral part of any meaningful experience - both painful and joyous. And by letting ourselves embrace these changes with strength and resilience, we can unlock the latent power within us to manifest our truest desires in life.

The Divine Union

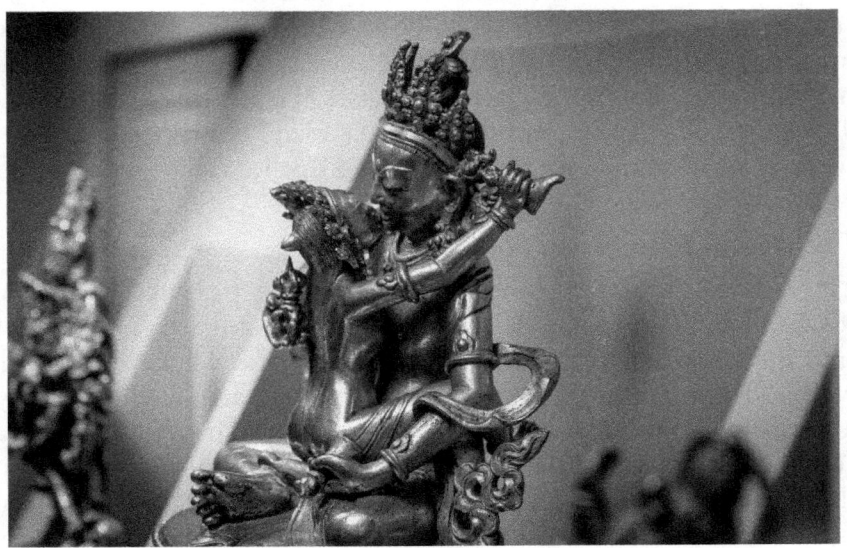

The Divine Union.
https://pixabay.com/es/photos/buda-tantra-estatua-shiva-shakti-4642497/

At the metaphysical level, Shiva and Shakti represent the divine union of male and female energy. In Hindu mythology, Shiva represents both the destructive and creative forces in the universe, while Shakti is the spiritual energy that animates life on earth. Together, they embody the perfect balance of masculine and feminine energy, essential for sustaining life. Through their intimate union, they create the dynamic cycle of creation and destruction that shapes our world.

By surrendering to this ever-changing dance of light and dark, we, too, can experience the profound peace that comes with acceptance and understanding. Whether you view them as mystical figures or symbols of inner wisdom, Shiva and Shakti remind us that every aspect of life is precious and worthy of our love and devotion. With their grace and guidance, we, too, can connect with this divine union within ourselves and embark on a journey toward liberation and fulfillment.

The Balance of Shakti and Shiva

Shakti and Shiva are intricately linked, sharing many qualities with each other. Although often viewed separately, as a pair, they form the perfect balance: while Shakti represents dynamic energy and action, Shiva represents stillness and reflection. Together, they create a harmonious equilibrium that allows the world to exist in perfect balance. And just as there can never be too much Shakti or too much Shiva, there can never be too much action or reflection - for these opposing forces together create an interconnected totality that is integral to everything that exists. So if we want to understand, protect, and appreciate the delicate balance of our world, we must first learn to value both Shakti and Shiva equally. After all, it is only by keeping them perfectly balanced that we can truly live in peace and harmony.

The Dance of Shakti and Shiva

The dance of Shakti and Shiva symbolizes the eternal union of opposites. Shiva represents transcendence and impermanence in this cosmic dance, while Shakti manifests as energy and change. Together, they embody the cyclical nature of life, constantly creating and destroying in a perpetual interplay of light and darkness. The dance itself also represents the ebb and flow of divine energy within ourselves. Just as we are buffeted by opposing forces in our day-to-day lives—struggling against setbacks even as we strive for success—we are always engaged in an inner struggle between our light and shadow selves. Ultimately, though, it is only by recognizing both sides that we can hope to achieve true balance, allowing us to tap into the infinite power projected by the Dance of Shakti and Shiva.

The Significance of Shakti and Shiva

When understanding the significance of Shakti and Shiva, perhaps the best place to start is with a basic understanding of their relationship. According to the ancient Hindu tradition, Shakti and Shiva are two halves of the same whole, perfectly matched in every way. Together they create a dynamic balance in all things and bring order to the universe. Moreover, from a more grounded perspective, Shakti and Shiva can be seen as representing two fundamental forces: energy and consciousness. Whether or not we are aware of them, these vital forces guide our thoughts, actions, and decisions daily. In this sense, Shakti and Shiva remind us that we contain both energy and consciousness within ourselves - and that through this understanding, we can find balance and greater fulfillment in our lives.

The Symbol of Shatkona

The shatkona is a powerful symbol revered by cultures worldwide for centuries. This enigmatic symbol holds a deep significance in Hindu and Buddhist traditions, representing the union of opposites in the world and on a spiritual level. Known as "the yoni of Devi," or goddess, this magical figure represents female fertility and abundance while simultaneously embodying peace and strength. Mystical in nature, the shatkona reminds us of the many paradoxes present in life and reminds us to embrace them all with open arms. Whether used in ritual or simply as a work of art, this complex symbol holds great meaning for anyone who seeks a deeper understanding of life.

The Purpose of Shakti and Shiva

Shakti and Shiva are at the heart of Hinduism, the divine forces of creation, preservation, and destruction. Shakti is often equated with the female creative energy of the universe, while Shiva is considered masculine personified. Together, these two deities symbolize the dynamic interplay between life and death principles that characterize existence. They are also responsible for maintaining a delicate balance within human nature: Shakti brings forth new life, while Shiva works to destroy it to pave the way for new beginnings. Through their union, Shakti and Shiva ultimately represent our ever-changing relationship with the cycles and seasons of life. And while they may seem paradoxical or even cruel at times, they remind us that change is at once both necessary and inevitable if we hope to grow and thrive in this world.

Shakti and Shiva are two of the most important deities in Hinduism, representing the forces of feminine and masculine energy. Shakti is often depicted as a goddess, embodying the power, dynamism, and creativity that lie at the heart of all natural things. Her counterpart, Shiva, represents stability, stillness, strength, and determination. Together, these energies act as a kind of cosmic dance – constantly changing and moving in response to each other to create balance. By understanding how these energies interact with each other and within ourselves, we can begin to glimpse the deeper mysteries of life itself. So whether you're seeking calm or creative inspiration, Shakti and Shiva can provide the tools you need to achieve your goals. With their timeless wisdom and transformative powers, they truly are two of the most important deities in the Hindu tradition.

Chapter 4: Samadhi: The Purpose of Meditation and Yoga

Have you ever achieved a state of complete absorption in something – so much so that time seems to stand still, and you are completely oblivious to your surroundings?

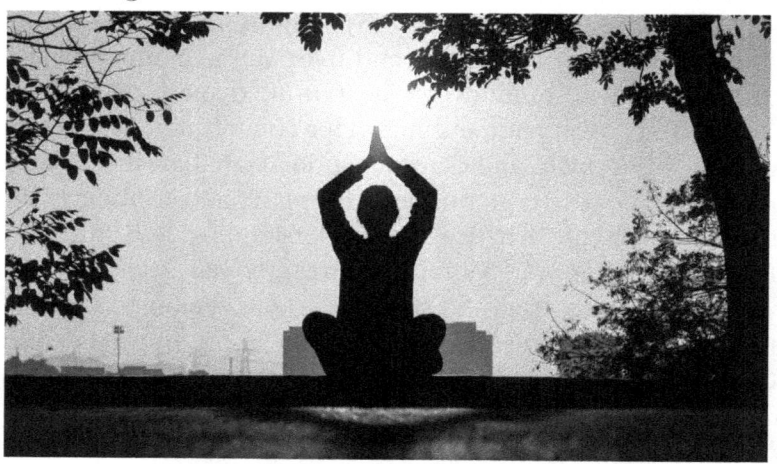

Yoga is a practice that encompasses every element of our being.
https://www.pexels.com/photo/silhouette-of-man-at-daytime-1051838/

Witnessing this state in others, we often label them as "in the zone" – they're completely engrossed in their actions. But this state is not unique to athletes or artists. Every one of us has experienced it at some point in our lives. This state is known as Samadhi in yoga and is considered the highest "limb" of Patanjali's "Eight Limbs of Yoga."

Yoga is not just a set of physical exercises to keep our bodies fit. It is a practice that encompasses every element of our being – physical, mental, emotional, and spiritual. The goal of yoga is to bring us into harmony with ourselves and the world around us. In this chapter, we will take a detailed look at Samadhi – what it is, its different levels, and how it can be achieved. We will also explore its relationship with Turiya and the various types of Samadhi. Finally, we will conclude with some tips and tricks that might help you on your journey to Samadhi.

Samadhi

The Sanskrit word for 'samadhi' comes from the root 'sam,' meaning to come together or concentrate. Samadhi, therefore, implies a state of complete absorption or single-pointed focus. It is a state in which the mind is completely still, and there is no sense of individual awareness. In this state, the subject and the object of meditation become one, and there is a sense of pure consciousness. When we are in a state of Samadhi, we are completely engrossed in what we are doing, and time seems to stand still. We are completely in the moment, and there is no room for any thoughts or distractions.

In Hinduism and Buddhism, Samadhi is often described as a superconscious state that is attained through meditation. Once we attain Samadhi, we see the world through the lens of our true nature – which is pure consciousness. From this state, we see things as they are, without the filters of our thoughts and emotions. This is why Samadhi is often described as a state of "no mind," where the mind is completely free from all thoughts.

The 8 Limbs of Yoga

The ancient spiritual and physical practice of yoga originated in India over 5000 years ago. The word *Yoga* comes from the Sanskrit root 'Yuj,' which means to yoke or unite. Yoga implies union – the union of the individual self with the universal self. This goal is achieved through the practice of the "Eight Limbs of Yoga," codified by the sage Patanjali in his text, the Yoga Sutras. These eight limbs guide us on our journey from the physical to the spiritual and from ignorance to enlightenment. While the first four limbs – the Yamas, Niyamas, Asanas, and Pranayamas – are designed to purify and prepare our bodies and minds for meditation, the last four – Pratyahara, Dharana, Dhyana, and Samadhi – are the actual stages of meditation. The practice of the first four limbs leads to developing the last four.

Yama

At the outset of your yoga practice, one of the first things you'll learn is Yama, the first limb of yoga. This concept consists of five core principles or ethical restraints, each focused on helping to cultivate a more compassionate and mindful way of living. The first principle, known as ahimsa or non-violence, encourages you to treat all living beings with kindness and consideration. This might mean being more mindful about how you eat, not harming animals in any way, and choosing not to participate in activities that cause harm or suffering.

The second principle of truthfulness helps you speak only the truth while avoiding even small white lies that might be harmful. Similarly, asteya or non-stealing encourages you to respect the rights and property of others, choosing not to take anything that does not belong to you without consent. The fourth principle, brahmacharya or chastity, focuses on creating healthy boundaries around your sexual behavior, encouraging self-control and integrity in all aspects of your life.

Finally, aparigraha –or non-possessiveness – promotes a balanced approach toward material wealth and encourages you to always prioritize what is most crucial in life – relationships and good health above everything else. Together these five principles form an essential foundation for all those who wish to embark on a journey toward greater wisdom and personal fulfillment through yoga. So if you're ready for change and growth in your life today, start with Yama – it will set you on the path towards achieving your goals both physically and mentally!

Niyama

In the second limb of yoga, known as Niyama, five positive duties form the basis of our practice. The first duty, Saucha or purity, refers to both physical and mental cleanliness and covers everything from healthy eating habits and regular physical activity to regular spiritual practice and meditation. Santosha or contentment refers to a sense of serenity and acceptance that arises when we cultivate gratitude for all we have. The third duty, Tapas or austerity, occupies a special place in the practice of yoga and is often viewed as a means for purifying ourselves through adversity and challenge.

Svadhyaya or self-study refers to the cultivation of introspection, reflection on our thoughts and actions, and self-reflection as a path towards gaining wisdom about who we are at our core. Finally, Ishvara Pranidhana, or surrendering ourselves to the will of Ishvara - otherwise known as God - serves as the ultimate act of inner transformation and understanding. Whether you are new to the practice of yoga or you have been practicing for many years, embracing these principles is sure to support your continued journey toward holistic well-being.

Asana

Asana is the third limb of yoga and refers to practicing physical postures or exercises. In many ways, this limb is unique compared to the other limbs of yoga. While the first two limbs involve practices such as meditation and focused breathing, asana is much more approachable for people who are new to the world of yoga. Unlike some of the more esoteric practices involved in other aspects of yogic life, asana involves simple movements that anyone of any level or familiarity with traditional yoga techniques can practice.

Incorporating asana into your practice can have many benefits, regardless of your level. These include improved flexibility and strength, increased energy levels, and deeper levels of concentration and awareness. Furthermore, by getting your body moving regularly through these gentle poses and stretches, you can help keep your immune system healthy too. So whether you are a newcomer to yoga or a seasoned practitioner looking to expand your horizons further, asana has something for everyone!

Pranayama

When practicing yoga, one of the key elements to focus on is your breathing. This, known as pranayama, involves regulating and controlling the flow of air in your body. By consciously slowing down your inhalations and exhalations, you can reach a sense of calm and inner focus. By paying attention to even the tiniest movements of breath within your body, you can become more attuned to the present moment. This way, pranayama is considered an essential part of any yoga regimen. So if you want to deepen your yoga practice and create greater health and well-being in your life, be sure to incorporate pranayama into your routine!

Pratyahara

Pratyahara is the fifth limb of yoga, which involves withdrawing one's senses from the outside world. This can be difficult for yoga practitioners, as we are constantly bombarded by sensory input from our surroundings. The goal of pratyahara, however, is to achieve control over these external stimuli to better focus inward. Through meditation, deep breathing exercises, and mindfulness training, yogis can learn to be aware of their inner experience while tuning out things like sounds, smells, sights, and physical sensations. Pratyahara ultimately helps us tap into our deepest inner selves and connect more profoundly with the world. So if you're interested in improving your sense of calm and inner focus through yoga practice, start with pratyahara!

Dharana

When practicing yoga, one of the critical components is Dharana: the ability to focus your mind and concentrate on a single task. This may involve focusing on the sensations in your body or attempting to clear your thoughts completely. Whatever your approach, the goal of Dharana is to cultivate mental clarity so that you can use your mind more effectively in both your yoga practice and other aspects of life.

Through regular practice, you'll begin to notice that it becomes easier and more natural for you to focus on one thing at a time without getting distracted by outside stimuli. Even when faced with challenges or difficult situations, you'll be better able to maintain your calm and composure by drawing on your Dharana skills. With time and deliberate practice, Dharana can help you become a stronger and more present version of yourself. Happy practicing!

Dhyana

Dhyana, or meditation, is the seventh limb of the path to enlightenment. This essential aspect of the tradition focuses on quieting the mind and body, helping practitioners to reach a state of calmness and completeness. With regular practice of Dhyana, one can become more mindful and gain a greater sense of self-understanding and awareness. This can profoundly impact one's life as a whole, allowing for deeper relationships with others, improved mental health, and greater emotional well-being. So whether you want to increase your focus and reduce stress or make progress on your spiritual journey, Dhyana is a powerful tool that can help you achieve these goals. So take some time today to try out this ancient practice for yourself and experience its many benefits!

Samadhi

Samadhi is the eighth and final limb of yoga, a practice that has been pursued for thousands of years. This state refers to the ultimate goal of many yoga practitioners: a superconscious state of full absorption or single-minded focus. In this state, one's thoughts become completely still, and one feels completely connected to the present moment. However, reaching Samadhi is not easy; it requires years of dedication and practice. Some believe this final stage can only be reached through deep meditation or intense physical discipline. While there are many different methods for achieving Samadhi, a commitment to exploring the inner world at a very deep level remains constant between all approaches. Through this journey, we come closer to understanding our true nature and connecting with our deepest sense of self.

Turiya and Samadhi

Turiya, or the fourth state of consciousness, refers to a highly elevated spiritual awareness thought to transcend both wakefulness and dreaming. This state can be accessed through various practices, including meditation and certain inward-focused yogic techniques. Samadhi, also known as bliss consciousness or enlightenment, is closely related to Turiya in that it involves a deep sense of oneness with the universe and all its inhabitants. Together, these states represent some of the highest forms of meditation to be achieved on this plane.

Turiya and Samadhi are often used interchangeably, but they are two different states. Turiya is a state of pure consciousness beyond normal waking, dreaming, and sleeping states. It is a state of pure awareness that is always present, even amidst the chaos of everyday life. On the other hand, Samadhi is a state of complete absorption in the present moment. It is a pure consciousness, free from thoughts or emotions. In Samadhi, the ego is completely dissolved, and one experiences a sense of oneness with the universe.

And while they are not easily attainable, those who reach them typically report feelings of intense peace and clarity, along with the experience of pure love for all living things. Thus, for those seeking spiritual growth through heightened consciousness, Turiya and Samadhi are truly transformative states that can offer deep insight into the nature of reality.

Levels of Samadhi

The concept of Samadhi can be a bit confusing for beginners since there are many different levels, and each one is distinct in its way.

Savikalpa Samadhi

There is much debate over the various levels of Samadhi, a meditative state characterized by a deep sense of peace and connection with the world. While many practitioners agree that there are ultimately three distinct levels – Savikalpa Samadhi, Nirvikalpa Samadhi, and Sahaja Samadhi – they often disagree on the details. For example, some believe that Savikalpa Samadhi can be further divided into two main levels: Samprajnata Samadhi and Asamprajnata Samadhi.

Samprajnata Samadhi is defined by a profound engagement with the world through perceptions, thoughts, and emotions. In other words, people in Samprajnata Samadhi still perceive the world around them and feel strong connections to their environment. This level is also sometimes referred to as Savikalpa Samadhi or Pratyaksa Anupratyaksa.

Asamprajnata Samadhi is a much deeper meditation in which all thoughts and sensory perceptions have completely faded. Rather than being engaged with the world through our senses or our thoughts, we become one with the underlying unity of all things in this final level of Savikalpa Samadhi. Ultimately, it is difficult to say definitively where one level ends and another begins because these states of consciousness are deeply subjective experiences that can look very different from one person to another. Regardless of these distinctions, both Samprajnata Samadhi and Asamprajnata Samadhi are considered powerful tools for connecting with our innermost selves and experiencing greater peace and harmony in our lives.

Nirvikalpa Samadhi

In many schools of yoga, Nirvikalpa Samadhi is the highest level of spiritual realization, and it marks a profound change in one's understanding of the nature of reality. This state of consciousness is characterized by complete absorption and a sense of oneness with the universe. During this state, the ego dissolves completely, freeing the practitioner to experience deep inner stillness and to commune directly with the source of all being. While achieving Nirvikalpa Samadhi may seem like an elusive goal for many yogis, those who dedicate themselves to this path will find that their hard work pays off in countless ways, both on and off the mat. Whether you are seeking spiritual fulfillment or simply a deeper sense of peace and calm within yourself, unlocking the power of Nirvikalpa Samadhi can transform your life in remarkable ways.

Sahaja Samadhi

At the highest level of Samadhi, there is a state of constant awareness known as Sahaja Samadhi. In this state, one can keep their focus on the divine presence even amid daily chaos. This ability comes from a deep sense of inner peace and equanimity, which allows one to remain centered even when faced with unexpected challenges or crises. To those who have reached this final level of Samadhi, life takes on a new sense of purpose and meaning. They know that with each moment that passes, they are slowly but surely advancing along their spiritual path and growing closer to true enlightenment. Whether running errands or dealing with difficult emotions, they know that it all simply contributes to their greater journey toward divinity. Thus, every second spent in awareness is truly precious for those who have reached this transcendent state of consciousness.

How to Achieve Samadhi

To achieve samadhi, *or a state of concentrated meditation*, you must first learn to quiet your mind and control your thoughts. This can be achieved through regular mindfulness practice or other focused breathing exercises. Once you have learned to calm your mind, you can begin to focus on one particular object or idea, such as the breath or a mantra. As you continue this practice, over time, you'll eventually enter into an intuitive state of consciousness known as samadhi. This deep meditative state can be used for several different purposes, from reading insights about yourself or the world around you to connecting spiritually with the universe. So if you are looking to achieve greater mental clarity and well-being, start by focusing on cultivating samadhi in your own life. With patience and dedication, you'll achieve this fulfilling state of meditation in no time.

Here are some tips for how to achieve Samadhi:

Practice

Practicing regularly to achieve samadhi and reach a deeper level of spiritual growth is crucial. Whether you take up meditation, chanting, or some other type of mindfulness exercise, regular practice is key to experiencing the true benefits of these activities. With consistent effort and patience, you'll gradually find yourself achieving greater levels of openness, clarity, and peace. And as you continue this mindful living path, you may eventually find yourself on the threshold of enlightenment itself.

Be Patient

It is critical to be patient and diligent in getting true peace of mind. Whether we are learning a new skill, working toward a challenging goal, or simply trying to maintain a healthy lifestyle, it takes time and consistency to cultivate the qualities that will support you on your journey to Samadhi. Patience is especially important when things get challenging or don't go as planned. Rather than giving up or getting discouraged, you should hold on to your intention with compassion and trust in yourself.

By being patient with ourselves and our circumstances, we can stay focused on the bigger picture and continue moving forward with confidence in our ability to succeed. As long as we keep doing our best every day and have faith in the journey, it is only a matter of time before we reach the state of calmness and serenity that we long for. So be patient: through consistent effort over time, you can find true happiness and fulfillment.

Surrender

Surrender is the key to achieving samadhi, a state of deep peace and equanimity that happens when we are fully present and connected to our true selves. At its essence, surrender means giving up our need to control and understand everything that happens around us. Instead, it involves letting go of ego-driven attachments and simply accepting what is. In doing so, we set aside the endless quest for empty happiness and satisfaction and instead open ourselves up to the experience of being fully alive. Over time, this deeper connection with our true selves allows us to live each moment from a place of profound stillness and acceptance, even amid intense challenges or difficulties. By surrendering to our experience with an open heart, we can gradually attain the liberating state of samadhi.

Detach

To achieve samadhi, or the state of deep meditation and connection with the universe, it is essential to learn how to detach from your thoughts and emotions. This is not an easy thing to do, especially if you are someone who tends to dwell too much on your problems and worries. However, learning how to detach gently from your experiences can help you cultivate a sense of calm that will help you to enter deep states of meditation more easily.

One effective way to begin detaching from your thoughts is simply by acknowledging them for what they are: fleeting mental events. As soon as a negative thought or emotion arises, take a step back from it. In other words, make yourself the silent observer of the thought or feeling rather than allowing yourself to fully engage with it. By taking this kind of detached approach toward your struggles, you'll gradually find it easier and easier to clear your mind and focus on connecting with the present moment. With practice, you may find that samadhi becomes almost effortless.

Witness

To reach the deepest state of relaxation and calmness, you need to first become a witness to your thoughts and sensations. This is often referred to as samadhi or enlightenment, and it can take a lot of time and effort to get to this level of awareness. However, with practice and dedication, it is possible to train your mind to enter this state at will.

Mindfulness meditation is a useful technique for developing awareness, where you simply allow your mind to be still and observe the thoughts that pass through without attaching meaning or judgment. This requires tremendous focus but can help you cultivate the mental clarity necessary for reaching samadhi. Additionally, you can also incorporate breathwork into your practice by focusing intently on every inhale and exhale. Paying close attention to how you breathe can create a sense of detachment from your thoughts and physical sensations, opening the door to a deeper level of consciousness.

With diligent work and an open mind, anyone can attain the state of samadhi and enjoy all the benefits that come with it. Whether you're looking for increased focus, reduced stress levels, or greater peace of mind, following these tips will help guide you down the path toward enlightenment.

Samadhi is a state of complete absorption in the present moment. It is a state of pure consciousness, free from any thoughts, emotions, or sense of self. The mind is completely still and at peace. Samadhi is the highest state that one can achieve in their yoga practice. It is a state of complete union with the universe. There are different levels of samadhi, from Savikalpa samadhi, a gateway to Turiya, to Nirvikalpa samadhi, the highest state of consciousness. To achieve samadhi, detach from your thoughts and emotions and become a witness of your mind. With practice and dedication, anyone can reach this state of complete peace and bliss.

Chapter 5: Yoga Poses That Pave the Way to Turiya

Yoga, this ancient Indian exercise method, can do wonders for your physical and mental health. On the physical side, yoga can help tone muscles, increase flexibility, and improve cardiovascular fitness. And from a mental standpoint, yoga can help to reduce stress levels, boost self-confidence, and increase overall well-being.

Whether you are just starting or have been practicing for many years, there is no question that yoga is a powerful tool for attaining Turiya. In this chapter, we will discuss some of the best yoga asanas or poses that can help you to reach this level of consciousness. We will also provide step-by-step instructions on how to get into each pose. Each of these asanas should be practiced regularly and can be done in the comfort of your own home.

Many different yoga asanas or poses can be beneficial for reaching Turiya. However, not all of them are suitable for beginners. We will focus on both challenging and beginner-friendly asanas that can still be quite effective. With regular practice, you'll progress to more advanced poses.

Tadasana - Mountain Pose

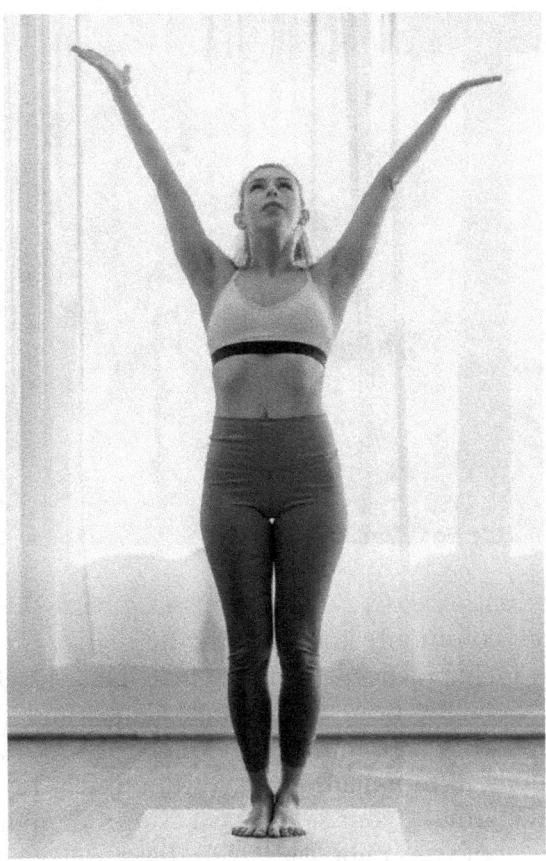

Mountain Pose.
https://www.pexels.com/photo/fit-woman-doing-tadasana-exercise-6453400/

Tadasana, or mountain pose, is a foundational posture in many forms of yoga. In this simple yet powerful posture, the body is balanced upright and rooted firmly to the ground, with all parts aligned in perfect symmetry. Starting with your feet hip-width apart, ground your feet into the floor and engage your leg muscles to firm your legs and kneecaps. Allow your rib cage to relax down as you lift through your spine, reaching gently upward towards the sky. Gaze forward with a soft focus or upward towards an imaginary point on the ceiling above you. Continuing to breathe deeply and evenly throughout the practice, hold tadasana for as long as feels comfortable. Slowly exhale at the end of each session and release back into a standing neutral posture before returning to your day.

Vrikshasana - Tree Pose

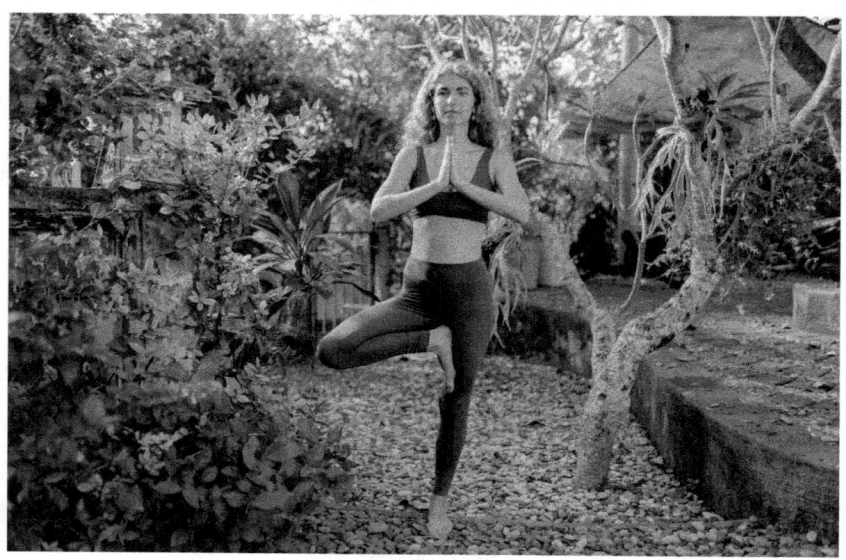

Tree Pose.
https://www.pexels.com/photo/a-woman-doing-yoga-in-the-garden-4457998/

Vrikshasana, more commonly known as the tree pose, is one of the most well-known and widely practiced yoga postures. This versatile posture has a wide range of benefits, from improving balance and coordination to strengthening the body's core muscles. To practice Vrikshasana, begin by setting up your body in mountain pose, with both feet firmly rooted into the ground and the arms at your sides. Next comes stepping your left foot about a foot in front of your right, with heels directly aligned.

After that, you can bring your hands together in a prayer position or place them on top of each other directly above your head. Finally, you root down through each foot and bend your supporting leg while lifting through the standing leg, holding this pose for five breaths before repeating it on the other side. With practice and patience, you'll find yourself mastering Vrikshasana and its many rewarding benefits!

Paschimottanasana - Seated Forward Bend

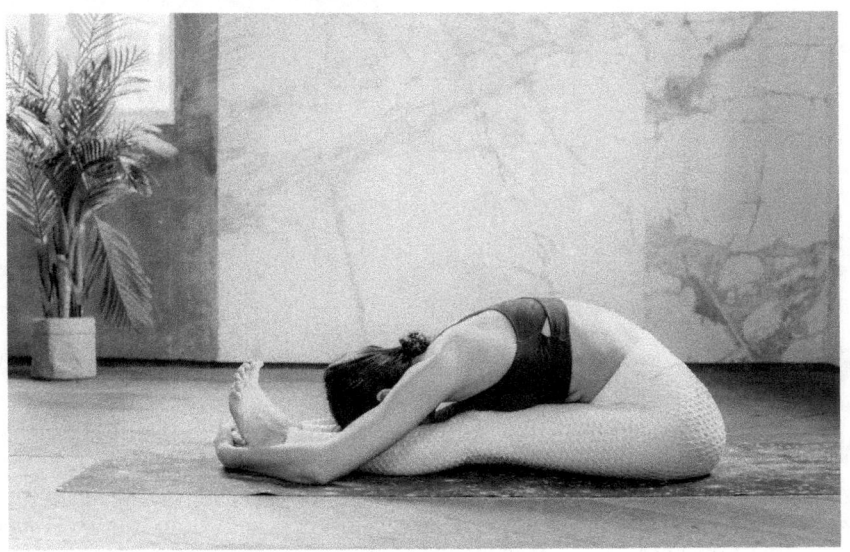

Seated Forward Bend.
https://www.pexels.com/photo/woman-practicing-yoga-3822191/

Paschimottanasana is a more advanced yoga pose that requires a lot of patience and practice to master. Although the name translates to "western forward bend," this posture can be done either standing or seated, depending on your current level of flexibility. To start, begin by sitting on the ground with your legs straight out in front of you. Make sure you're sitting comfortably with your back supported by a cushion or chair.

Next, slowly fold forward at the hips, trying to bring your chest as close as possible to your thighs. As you do so, focus on keeping your back flat and lengthening through the spine. Finally, once you've reached your maximum range of motion for this pose, hold the position for 30 seconds or longer if possible. Repeat this process regularly until you've mastered the pose and can comfortably hold it for five minutes or more at a time. With persistence and dedication, anyone can gain the strength and flexibility necessary to successfully perform Paschimottanasana!

Halasana - Plow Pose

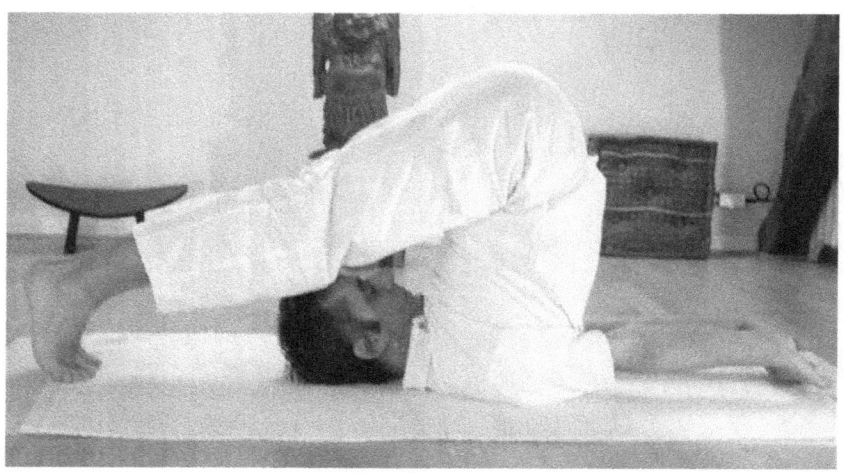

Plow Pose.

Joseph RENGER, CC BY-SA 3.0 <http://creativecommons.org/licenses/by-sa/3.0/>, via Wikimedia Commons: https://commons.wikimedia.org/wiki/File:Halasana.jpg

Halasana, also known as Plow Pose, is a classic yoga posture designed to stretch and strengthen the entire body. This pose primarily strengthens and stretches the core, legs, and back. When performed correctly, Halasana helps to elongate and tone the spine's natural curves while building core strength. Additionally, this pose has been shown to improve circulation and digestion while reducing stress and fatigue.

To practice Halasana, begin by lying flat on your back with your legs extended straight in front of you. Next, slowly lift your legs over your head, keeping your back flat on the ground and your knees straight. Once your legs are in line with your body, allow them to fall over towards the floor behind you, using your hands to support your lower back if necessary. Finally, once you're in the full plow position, focus on deep breathing and hold the pose for as long as possible. When you're ready to come out of the pose, slowly roll your back onto the floor and bring your legs back to their starting position. With regular practice, you'll be able to hold this pose for five minutes or more at a time!

Sarvangasana - Shoulder Stand

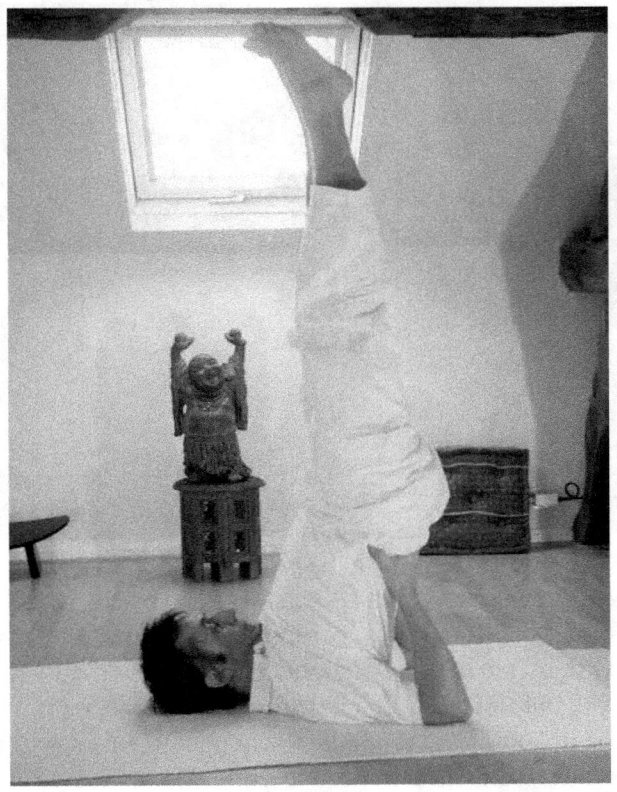

Shoulder Stand.
Joseph RENGER, CC BY-SA 3.0 <http://creativecommons.org/licenses/by-sa/3.0/>, via Wikimedia Commons: https://commons.wikimedia.org/wiki/File:Sarvangasana.jpg

Sarvangasana, also known as the shoulder stand, is an asana that has been practiced for millennia by yogis and yoginis alike. This pose is believed to offer a wide range of health benefits, from improved circulation and digestion to relief from stress and anxiety. To perform Sarvangasana properly, one must begin by lying flat on their back with feet close together. From there, the practitioner will then gently lift their legs into the air using their shoulders as support. Finally, they will hold this position for several breaths, paying careful attention to maintain proper alignment in the rest of their body throughout the pose. Whether you are a beginner or an advanced practitioner, Sarvangasana is sure to be a valuable addition to your yoga practice.

Setu Bandhasana - Bridge Pose

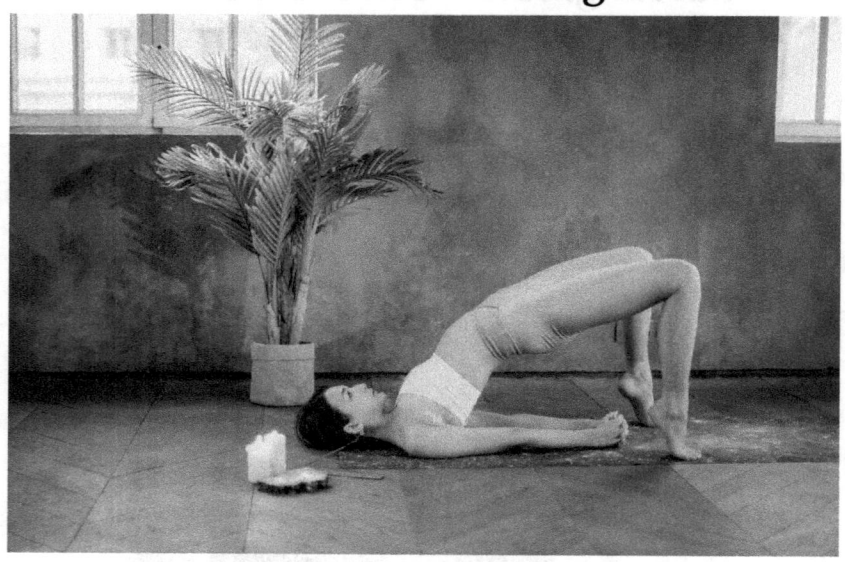

Bridge Pose.
https://www.pexels.com/photo/woman-practicing-yoga-3822650/

Setu Bandhasana, also known as Bridge Pose, is a crucial yoga pose that helps to strengthen the lower back and core. To perform this pose, you first need to lie flat on your back with your knees bent and your feet pressed into the ground. Next, you'll slowly raise your hips towards the sky until your shoulders are directly above your pelvis and your upper body forms a straight line from head to tailbone. At this point, engaging all of your core muscles is important to maintain proper form throughout the entire pose. You can hold Bridge Pose for any desired length of time or repeat it multiple times as part of an overall yoga routine. With regular practice, Setu Bandhasana can help to improve posture and overall flexibility, making it a great way to start or end any yoga session.

Matsyasana - Fish Pose

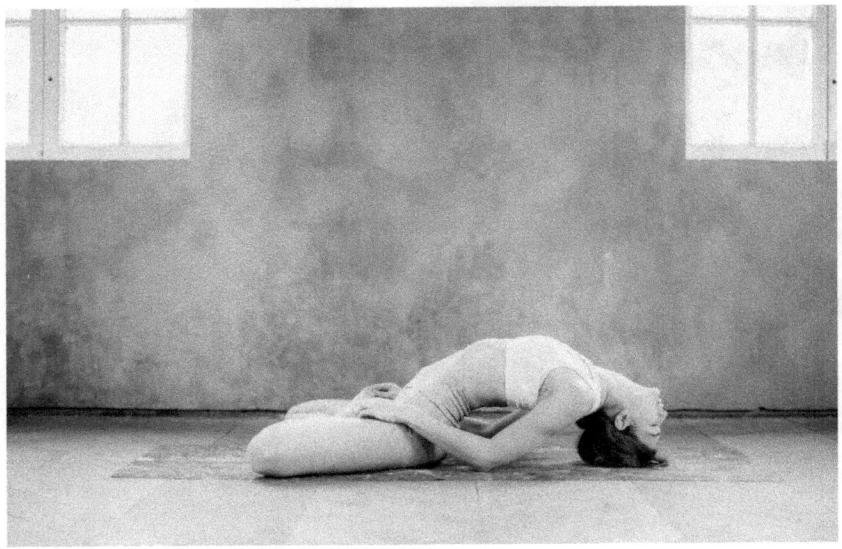

Fish Pose.
https://www.pexels.com/photo/woman-practicing-yoga-3822585/

Matsyasana, or Fish Pose, is a powerful yoga posture that can help to open up your spine and stretch your core. This pose requires you to lie flat on your back and rest your body weight on your upper chest and head. To enter the pose, simply fold your legs towards the torso, arch your back slightly upward, and press your hands into the floor behind you for support.

Once you're in the proper position, you can start to pay attention to the sensations in your body, breathing deeply as you hold the position. With practice, this relaxing and rejuvenating posture can help to improve flexibility and strengthen core muscles, making it a great tool for improving overall health and well-being. Whether used alone or as part of a comprehensive practice, Matsyasana is an essential pose for anyone who wants to harness the power of yoga.

Uttanasana - Standing Forward Bend

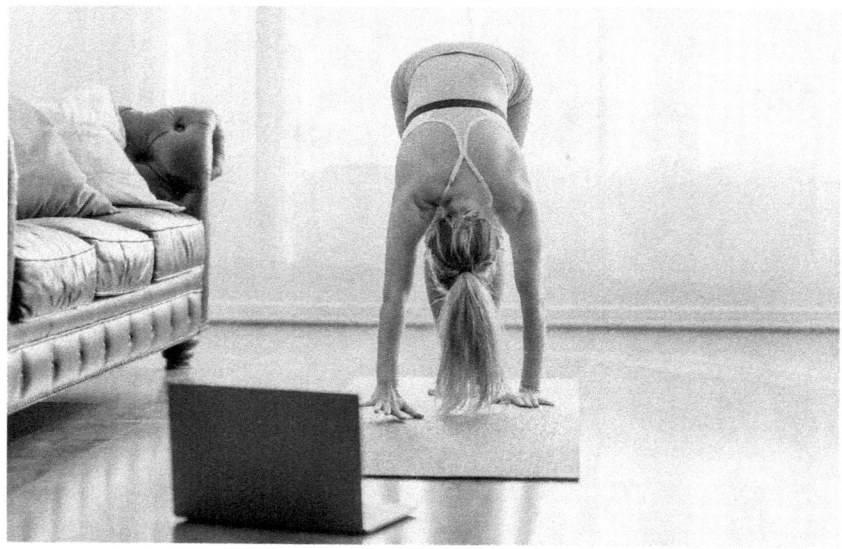

Standing Forward Bend.
https://www.pexels.com/photo/anonymous-fit-woman-doing-uttanasana-posture-6453398/

Uttanasana, or the standing forward bend, is a powerful yoga pose that offers a wide range of benefits. From improving posture and flexibility to relieving stress and anxiety, this simple yet effective pose can do wonders for both the body and mind. To practice Uttanasana, begin by standing with your feet hip-width apart and your hands at your sides. Next, hinge forward at the hips until you are in a flat tabletop position with your hands planted firmly on the floor in front of you. Slowly walk your hands forward until they are fully extended while keeping your hips firmly rooted to the ground. Breathe deeply as you hold this pose for several seconds or longer if desired. When ready, slowly rise back up to a standing position, feeling all of the wonderful benefits that Uttanasana has to offer.

Ardha Matsyendrasana - Half Spinal Twist

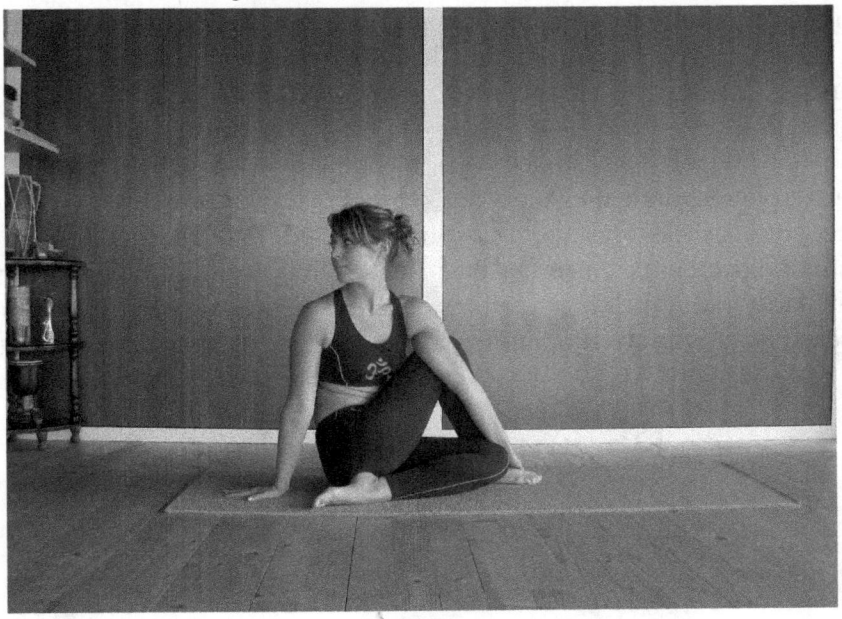

Half Spinal Twist.

Iveto, CC BY-SA 4.0 <https://creativecommons.org/licenses/by-sa/4.0>, via Wikimedia Commons: https://commons.wikimedia.org/wiki/File:Ardha-Matsyendrasana1.JPG

Ardha Matsyendrasana, or the Half Spinal Twist, is a popular yoga pose renowned for its many health benefits. This inverted pose gently stretches and opens up the spine, allowing you to release any built-up tension in your back. It also stimulates and massages the organs of the abdominal region, helping to regulate digestion. Additionally, this pose can help to improve balance and stability, making it an excellent choice for anyone looking to increase their flexibility and overall fitness level.

The procedure for performing Ardha Matsyendrasana is relatively simple. To begin, sit on the ground with your legs extended in front of you. Then, bring your right foot to rest on the ground next to your left thigh. Complete the pose by twisting your body to the right and stretching your left hand to the ground behind you. Breathe deeply and hold this pose for several seconds before repeating it on the other side. With regular practice, Ardha Matsyendrasana can help to improve your flexibility, reduce stress and anxiety, and promote overall physical and mental well-being.

Pasasana - Noose Pose

Pasasana, or the Noose Pose, is a powerful and challenging yoga posture that requires focus, strength, and flexibility. To perform this asana, you begin in a sitting position with your legs crossed and your arms outstretched over your head. Next, you bend forward from the waist and reach for one of your ankles with each hand. You then draw the feet toward yourself until the heels are close to or even touching your hips. Once you have established this position, you may hold it for several breaths before gently releasing back to a sitting position. This posture is particularly helpful for stretching and strengthening the lower body muscles. So if you are looking for a challenge in your next yoga practice, give Pasasana a try!

Dhanurasana - Bow Pose

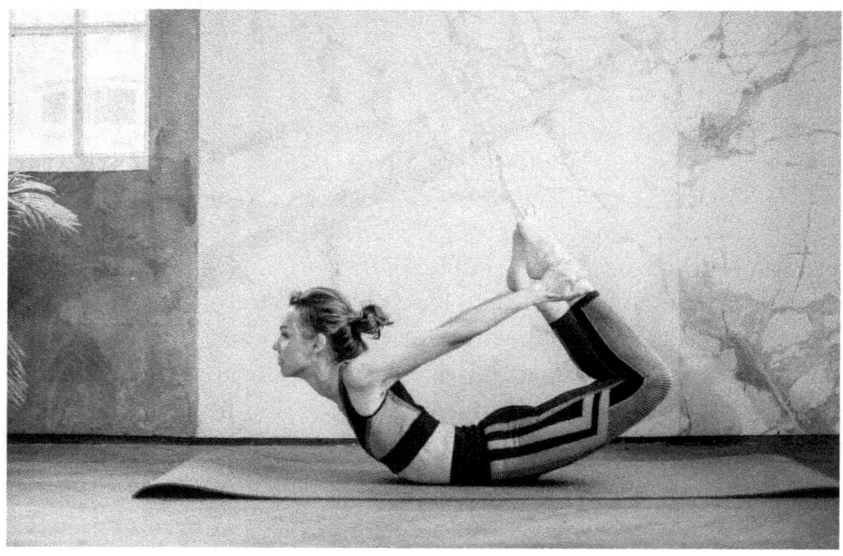

Bow Pose.
https://www.pexels.com/photo/woman-bow-pose-3822366/

Dhanurasana, also known as the *bow pose*, is a powerful yoga posture that can provide plenty of benefits for your body and mind. This pose works to stretch and strengthen the muscles in the abdominal region, including the lower back and core muscles. It also helps to improve circulation and digestion, making it a great way to start your day or break up a longer yoga session. Additionally, this pose encourages focus, breath control, and balance while helping you to relieve stress and anxiety.

To perform dhanurasana, or *bow pose*, begin by lying flat on your stomach with your arms by your sides. Next, reach back and grab hold of your ankles with your hands. Slowly lift your chest and legs off of the ground, using your abdominal muscles to stay lifted. Breathe deeply and hold this position for several seconds or longer if desired. To release, gently lower your body back to the ground and relax. With regular practice, you'll soon be enjoying all of the benefits that Dhanurasana has to offer!

Ustrasana - Camel Pose

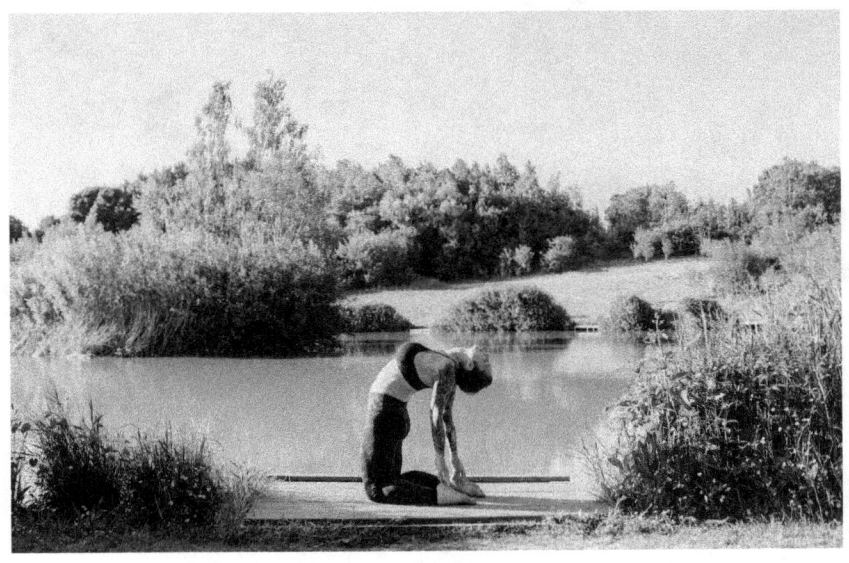

Camel Pose
https://www.pexels.com/photo/flexible-woman-performing-camel-pose-on-dock-against-lake-4793286/

At first glance, Ustrasana might seem like a fairly straightforward yoga pose. This posture calls for you to get down on your hands and knees, with your knees hip-width apart, and slowly arch or extend your spine upward. As you extend, you should reach back along the inside of your legs until you can clasp the outer thighs or heels if possible. Hold this position for a few breaths, then release back to starting position.

While it may seem easy at first, Ustrasana requires a great deal of balance and strength as well as flexibility in both the hips and back. To help prepare yourself for this challenging pose, start with some warm-up exercises that gently stretch and open up the hips and lower back. These will help you enter into Ustrasana with more stability and less risk of injury. With time and practice, however, this powerful posture can help you tap into your full potential and unlock new levels of strength, flexibility, and focus.

Bhujangasana - Cobra Pose

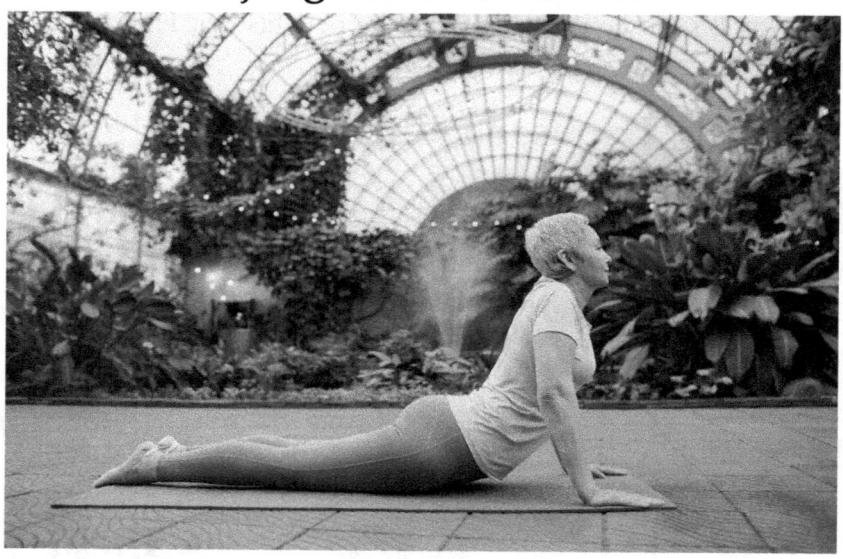

Cobra Pose.
https://www.pexels.com/photo/woman-doing-cobra-pose-6787216/

Bhujangasana, also known as the cobra pose, is one of the most popular yoga postures for both beginners and advanced practitioners. This back-bending pose helps to stretch and strengthen the major muscles in the lower back while gently mobilizing the spine. It can also improve circulation, relieve stress, and increase flexibility. To enter into Bhujangasana, start by lying down with your stomach on the ground and your legs extended straight behind you. Next, place your hands palm-down on the ground beside your shoulders. Slowly begin to lift your head and chest off the ground, using your back muscles to support you. Gaze upward and hold this position for a few breaths before releasing it back down to the starting position. With regular practice of Bhujangasana, you can reap all of its many benefits and enjoy improved overall health and well-being.

Salabhasana - Locust Pose

Salabhasana, or Locust Pose, is a powerful yoga pose used to build strength and flexibility throughout the body. To perform this pose, you first lie on your stomach with your arms at your sides and press firmly through your hands and feet. Next, raise your head, chest, and legs off of the ground while keeping your core engaged in maintaining balance. Hold this pose for a few deep breaths before returning to the starting position, taking care to fully relax muscles and joints as you come down. Overall, Salabhasana is an excellent practice for improving strength and flexibility in the back, shoulders, and abdomen muscles. Whether you are a beginner just starting or an experienced yogi looking to deepen your practice, Salabhasana has something to offer everyone!

Uttar Pradesh Asana - Upward Plank Pose

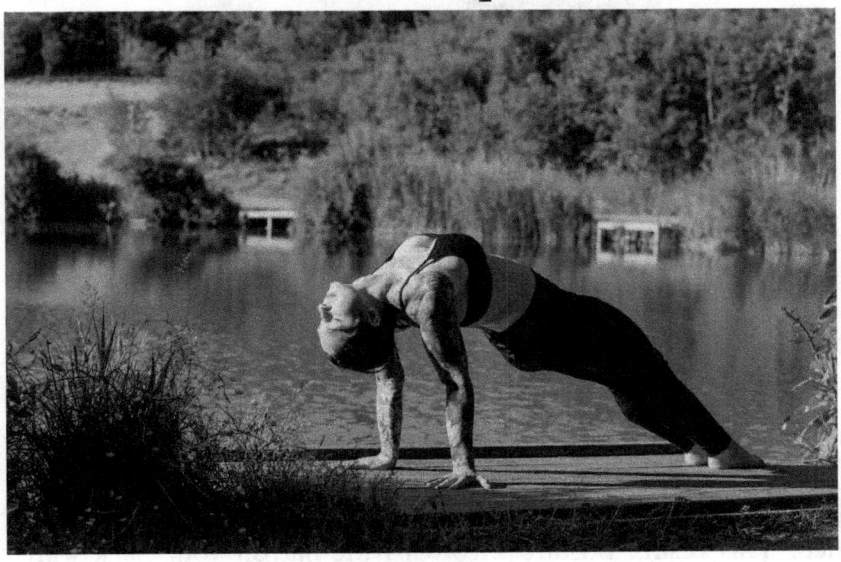

Upward Plank Pose.
https://www.pexels.com/photo/flexible-tattooed-woman-standing-in-upward-plank-pose-4793284/

The Uttar Pradesh Asana is a challenging yoga pose that requires both flexibility and strength. One of the key advantages of this pose is that it helps to build upper body strength, particularly in the shoulders, arms, and torso. To perform it, you'll start by lying flat on your stomach with your legs together and your arms extended out in front of you. You then used your hands to push yourself up into an elevated plank position with straight arms and flexed feet. From here, you'll hold the position for several seconds before gently lowering yourself back down to the ground. With regular practice, this asana can help improve overall strength and blood flow throughout the body. So if you're looking for a new challenge in your yoga practice, give the Uttar Pradesh Asana a try.

Shavasana - Corpse Pose

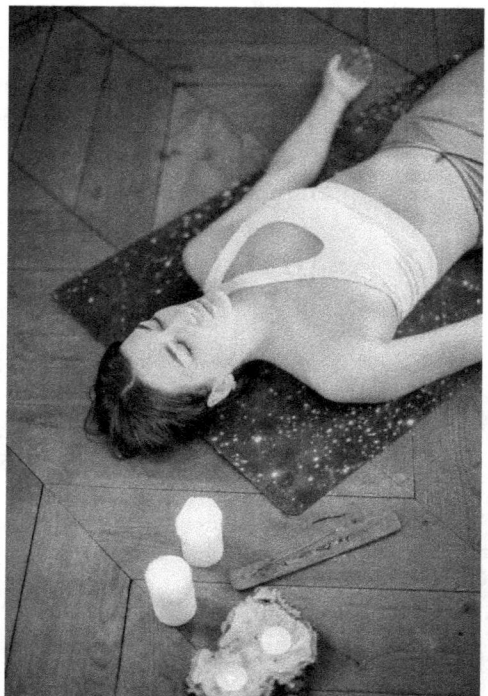

Corpse Pose.
https://www.pexels.com/photo/woman-relaxing-in-yoga-mat-3822647/

Shavasana, or the corpse pose, is one of the essential elements of any yoga practice. This restful posture involves lying flat on your back with your arms and legs spread wide, releasing all tension and stress from your body. Not only does Shavasana help to relax the physical body, but it also allows you to calm your mind and reflect on your thoughts and feelings in a more grounded way. Many yogis claim that spending just a few minutes in this pose every day helps them improve their overall well-being and reconnect with themselves on a deeper level. Seen as a way to relax and rejuvenate, Shavasana is an essential pose for anyone looking to improve their health and well-being.

Viparita Karani - Legs up the Wall Pose

Viparita Karani, or Legs Up the Wall Pose, is a simple but effective yoga pose that is great for revitalizing the body and calming the mind. This posture involves lying on the floor with your legs elevated against a wall, either straight up or at an angle. The key to this pose is keeping the spine long and flat as your legs move upward. This helps to stretch out and decompress the lower back, which makes it an excellent remedy for tightness and soreness in this area. At the same time, Viparita Karani also helps to calm and soothe the nervous system by stimulating blood circulation throughout the body. So if you're looking for a quick way to feel more energized and balanced, try practicing this simple yet powerful pose!

Adho Mukha Svanasana - Downward Facing Dog Pose

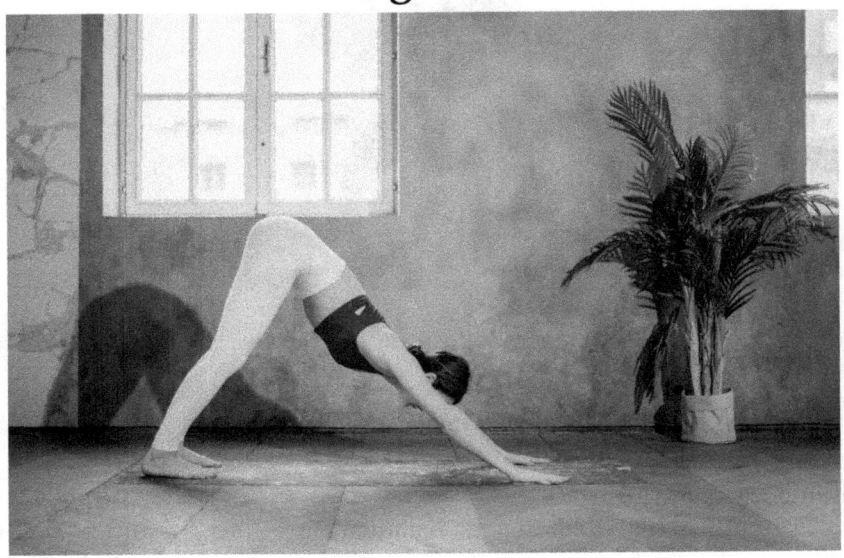

Downward Facing Dog Pose.
https://www.pexels.com/photo/woman-in-downward-dog-pose-3822118/

Adho Mukha Svanasana, commonly known as the Downward Facing Dog Pose, is one of the most popular yoga poses in practice today. This powerful pose can be challenging at first, as it requires strength, flexibility, and balance to hold it properly. However, with regular practice, this incredible posture can help to build strength and flexibility throughout your entire body while also increasing blood flow and circulation. Additionally, Adho Mukha Svanasana is great for improving posture and relieving stress, making it a must-have tool for any yoga routine.

To give the Downward Facing Dog Pose a try, start in a tabletop position on your hands and knees with your wrists under your shoulders and your knees under your hips. From here, lift your hips up and back, straightening your legs as you move into an inverted "V" position. Keep your core engaged and your breath steady as you hold the pose for several seconds. With regular practice, you'll develop the strength and flexibility needed to hold this pose for longer periods.

Bakasana - Crow Pose

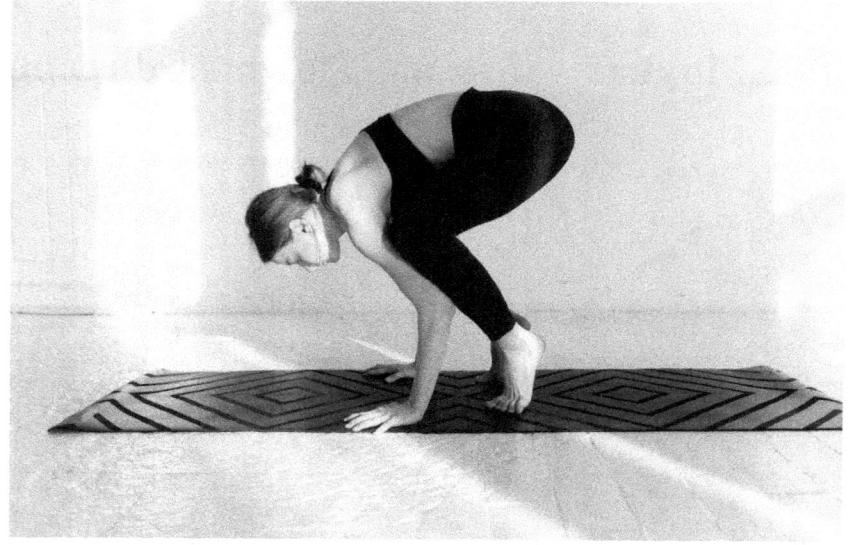

Crow Pose.
https://www.pexels.com/photo/a-woman-doing-a-crow-pose-6739072/

Bakasana, also known as Crow Pose, is one of the most popular yoga poses around. This challenging balancing posture requires strength, flexibility, and focus, making it a popular go-to pose for yogis looking to challenge their bodies and mind. To enter Bakasana, start in a standing position with your feet about hip-width apart. Coming down into a low squat on your toes, shift your weight into your hands and begin to bend your arms. Then, place your knees on the back of your upper arms and slowly start to lift your hips off the ground. The key to this pose is to keep your core engaged and your breath steady as you maintain your balance.

With practice, you can gradually lower yourself down onto your forearms to deepen the pose and increase the challenge. Whether you are a beginner or an experienced practitioner, Bakasana is sure to leave you feeling strong, flexible, and focused!

Virabhadrasana - Warrior Pose

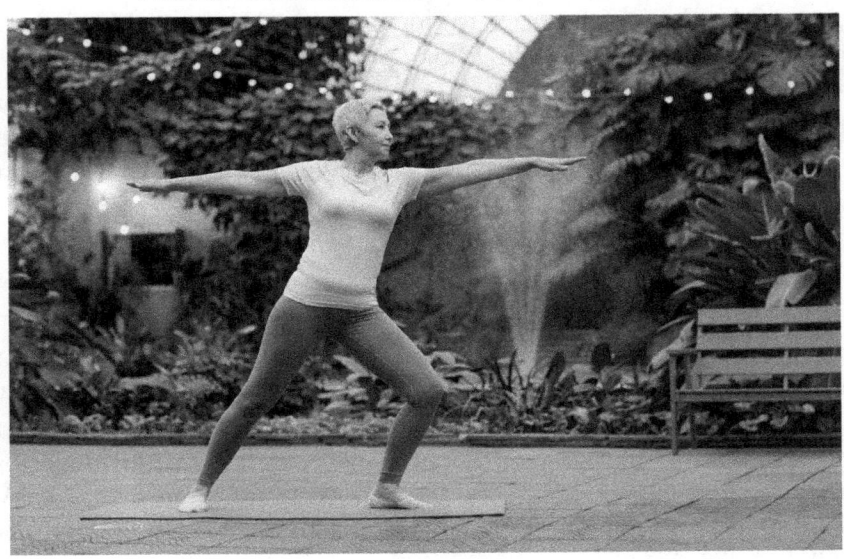

Warrior Pose.
https://www.pexels.com/photo/woman-doing-warrior-pose-6787161/

Virabhadrasana, also known as Warrior Pose, is a powerful and dynamic yoga posture renowned for building strength and stamina. To perform this pose, begin in a standing position with your feet about hip-width apart. Step your left foot back and angle it out to the side so that your toes are pointing outward at a 45-degree angle. At the same time, bring your right arm up and overhead, keeping your palm facing inward toward your body. Then, lift your right knee so that your thigh is parallel to the ground and your knee is directly above your ankle. Hold this position for several deep breaths before releasing and repeating on the other side. With regular practice, you'll develop the strength and stamina needed to hold this pose for longer periods. With proper alignment, this posture can help to tone the legs and strengthen the core. Additionally, this pose promotes flexibility in the hips and upper body and increases blood flow throughout the body.

Putting It All Together

Now that we've explored the basics of yoga and some popular individual poses, it's time to put those moves together into a complete routine. Depending on your level of experience, you can start with a long flow, gradually working up to more advanced postures as you go. Some of the best, most fundamental poses to include are Downward-Facing Dog, Warrior pose, as well as Standing Forward Bend.

Whether you're focusing on strength or flexibility, these basic movements will help you build a strong foundation in your yoga practice. And with regular practice and dedication, you'll find yourself becoming stronger and more balanced – both on and off the mat. Remember, there is no one "right" way to do yoga. The key is to find what works best for you and to go at your own pace.

Yoga is a great way to improve your health and well-being. With regular practice, you can experience increased strength and flexibility, improved balance and posture, and decreased stress levels. Whether you're new to yoga or have been practicing for years, there are always new things to learn and explore on the mat. While there are many different individual poses, begin by including the most fundamental poses in your practice. With dedication and commitment, you can develop a strong foundation in yoga that will help improve your overall health and quality of life.

So there you have it! A beginner's guide to yoga, complete with illustrations and step-by-step instructions. With regular practice, you'll develop the strength, flexibility, and balance needed to progress in your yoga journey. And who knows? You might even find yourself achieving Turiya along the way.

Chapter 6: Using Pranayama to Induce Turiya

Since the dawn of time, people have been striving to find ways to improve their lives and attain a higher state of consciousness. In recent years, there has been a resurgence of interest in ancient practices such as yoga and meditation, which have numerous benefits for both the mind and body. Among the many different techniques used in yoga and meditation, pranayama (breath control) is said to be particularly effective in attaining a higher state of consciousness, known as Turiya.

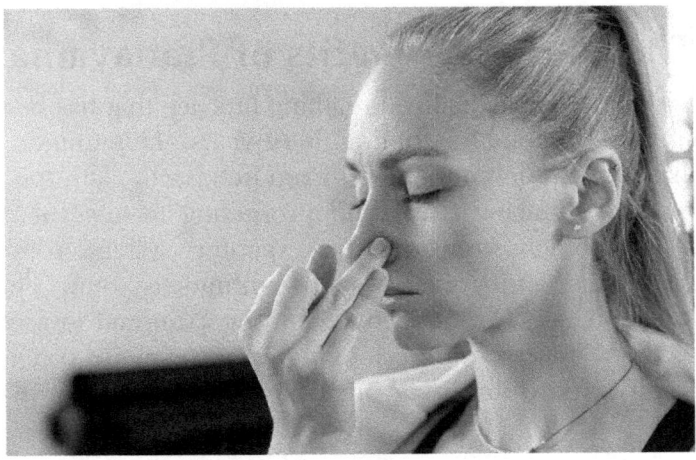

Pranayama is said to be particularly effective in attaining a higher state of consciousness, known as Turiya.
https://www.pexels.com/photo/a-woman-doing-nostril-breathing-6648567/

This chapter will explore the benefits of pranayama, both scientific and spiritual, and how it can help in attaining Turiya. We will also introduce the concept of "prana" and explore different types of pranayama techniques that can be used to achieve Turiya. By the end of this chapter, you should have a better understanding of how pranayama can help you achieve Turiya and some of the different techniques that you can use to reach this state.

Pranayama's Role in Achieving Turiya

Pranayama is an essential element of yogic practice, helping to cultivate mental and physical clarity. In Sanskrit, the word pranayama means "restriction of breath" or "control of breath," referring to the act of controlling one's breathing to achieve states of deeper awareness. Through proper control and concentration on the breath, yogis can achieve turiya, the deep meditative state that brings about a profound sense of peace and well-being.

Pranayama is also known for its therapeutic effects, helping to relieve stress and anxiety while also increasing energy levels and reducing inflammation. Whether you are new to yoga or a long-time practitioner, pranayama has much to offer in terms of cultivating greater wisdom and understanding. So why not give it a try? With regular practice, you might just find yourself enjoying all the benefits that this powerful breathing technique has to offer.

The Various Benefits of Pranayama

Pranayama is a type of meditative breathing practice that has been used in various spiritual traditions for thousands of years. This unique breathing technique has many different benefits, from helping to calm the mind and increase focus to reducing stress and promoting feelings of well-being. Pranayama can also help strengthen the respiratory system, improve blood flow to vital organs, and even boost the immune system. This ancient practice has also been shown to reduce chronic pain and improve overall physical health. Whether you are looking for an effective way to manage stress or simply want to improve your overall health, pranayama is a tool that is worth exploring.

Scientific Benefits of Pranayama
1. Pranayama and the Nervous System

Pranayama has long been used to calm and balance the nervous system. This ancient practice involves cultivating control over the breath, allowing us to develop greater awareness of our body and mind. By bringing attention to the subtle sensations associated with each inhalation and exhalation, we learn to better regulate both our breath and our internal states. And by focusing on the mental effects of pranayama, we can begin to see how the incessant chatter of our mind affects our overall well-being. Through these practices, pranayama helps us to stay grounded and present in the face of stress, anxiety, and other overwhelming emotions. Overall, this ancient technique offers a powerful way to support and heal our minds and bodies by tapping into the very foundation of who we are: our breath.

2. Pranayama and the Respiratory System

Pranayama is an essential component of many traditional approaches to respiratory health. This ancient practice works by consciously controlling one's breath, expanding and contracting the diaphragm as air moves in and out of the lungs, thereby calming and focusing the mind. Practitioners believe that this slow, rhythmic breathing regulates both the prana, or vital life force, and the nadis (or channels) that carry information throughout the body. And while the effects of this powerful breathing technique have been largely anecdotal until now, new research has revealed that pranayama can significantly impact respiratory function and overall well-being.

Studies by the National Institute of Mental Health and Neurosciences (NIMHANS) in India have shown that pranayama can help to improve airflow to the lungs, reduce bronchial congestion, and increase overall lung capacity. In addition, this traditional practice has been shown to improve blood oxygenation and help to alleviate asthma and other respiratory conditions. Controlled breathing can also improve lung capacity, regulate respiratory rate and rhythm, relieve stress and anxiety, relieve sleep apnea symptoms, improve cardiovascular function, and even reduce coughing due to smoke exposure. By harnessing the power of pranayama, we can all experience these incredible benefits for ourselves, improving our mental clarity, physical strength, and overall sense of well-being.

3. Pranayama and the Cardiovascular System

Studies by the National Institute of Mental Health and Neurosciences (NIMHANS) in India have shown that pranayama can be especially good for the cardiovascular system, improving circulation and reducing blood pressure. This is due in part to the indirect effects of yogic breathing, including lowered stress levels and increased relaxation. Additionally, pranayama itself may help to release nitric oxide into the bloodstream, which increases blood flow and helps to open up blocked arteries. Overall, pranayama is an excellent tool for keeping your heart healthy and strong, so it's worth incorporating into your daily routine.

4. Pranayama and the Digestive System

Pranayama, or controlled breathing, has many known benefits for the body and mind. Not only does it help to relieve stress and anxiety, but it can also enhance physical health, especially when it comes to the digestive system. Pranayama increases the production of digestive juices, improves digestion, and relieves constipation. Additionally, regular practice of pranayama techniques improves digestion and improve overall gut health by increasing blood circulation, stimulating healthy bacteria growth, reducing inflammation, and supporting immune function. Because of these potent effects on the digestive system, Pranayama is an essential tool for anyone looking to optimize their gut health and improve their overall well-being. So if you're dealing with a chronic gut issue or simply want to feel more energized throughout the day, incorporating pranayama into your daily routine is a great way to start. With just ten or fifteen minutes of practice per day, you can begin reaping all of the rewards that this ancient breathing technique has to offer.

5. Pranayama and the Immune System

Pranayama is a form of yoga that focuses on breathing exercises to help promote good health. One of the primary benefits of pranayama is its impact on the immune system. By stimulating certain organs and glands in the body, pranayama actively supports the immune system in its work of fighting off viruses, bacteria, and other toxins. In addition, pranayama also helps to reduce stress and anxiety, both of which have been shown to weaken our defenses against illness. Through regular practice of pranayama, it is possible to support our bodies in all aspects of wellness, from physical health to mental clarity. Ultimately, this makes pranayama one of the best ways to boost immunity and maintain overall well-being.

Spiritual Benefits of Pranayama
1. Pranayama and the Mind

By consciously controlling our breath, we can direct vital energy (or prana) throughout our body. This can have several mental and emotional benefits, including enhanced focus, reduced stress, and improved moods. This practice also promotes relaxation and inner calmness, helping us connect more deeply with the present moment. Pranayama also activates certain areas of the brain associated with meditation; in other words, it functions as a type of 'spiritual bypass,' allowing us to tap into deeper states of consciousness within ourselves. Thus, pranayama is an essential part of any well-rounded yoga or meditative practice. With regular practice, you can reap all the benefits that this gentle yet transformative breath work has to offer.

2. Pranayama and the Body

While Pranayama has traditionally been seen as a form of meditation and personal spiritual transformation, more recent research has shown that pranayama also offers numerous physical benefits. For example, studies have found that regular pranayama practice can strengthen the respiratory system, improve circulation, and help to relieve stress and anxiety. Pranayama also helps to improve focus and concentration, helping us to feel more energized and balanced throughout the day. So if you are looking for a powerful way to enhance your health and well-being, consider incorporating some pranayama into your practice today. You won't regret it!

3. Pranayama and the Spirit

Pranayama is more than just a breathing exercise; it is a powerful spiritual and physical practice with many benefits. Consciously controlling your breath can help you become more aware of your body and mind. In addition, the calming effect of deep, rhythmic breaths reduces feelings of tension and nervousness, making pranayama an excellent tool for promoting mental well-being. On a deeper level, pranayama is said to help connect you with your highest self or spirit. Through concentration and focused breathing, you can feel yourself becoming more centered, clear-minded, and calm. Overall, pranayama offers countless benefits for the body, mind, and spirit – making it one of the most powerful practices in yoga and general life.

An Introduction to the Concept of "Prana"

Prana is an ancient concept that has played an essential role in various spiritual traditions throughout history. Often referred to as the "breath of life," prana refers to the vital energy that surrounds and permeates everything in the universe. This includes living things and inanimate objects like rocks, rivers, and even entire planets.

While prana may seem somewhat intangible, it is considered a crucial part of any functioning system – from a single-celled organism to the entire cosmos. In the yogic tradition, prana is thought to be the life force that animates and sustains all living beings. It flows through the body in a network of energy channels called nadis. There are 72,000 nadis in total, with three main channels running along the spine: the Ida (left), Pingala (right), and Sushumna (central). The breath is a direct manifestation of prana, and the practice of pranayama is one of the most effective ways to harness this life-giving energy. By controlling the breath, we can control the flow of prana within the body and use it to our advantage.

Different Types of Pranayama Techniques

While the technique of pranayama may seem simple enough – after all, it is just breath control – there are many different ways to practice this art. Here are a few of the most popular pranayama techniques that you can try today:

1. Nadi Shodhana

Nadi Shodhana Pranayama, or alternate nostril breathing, is yet another popular yoga technique beneficial for the body and mind. This ancient breathing practice involves breathing in through one nostril at a time, calming the nerves and improving concentration. To begin practicing Nadi Shodhana Pranayama, start by sitting comfortably with your back straight but not rigid. You can also choose to lie down if you prefer. Close your eyes and focus on taking slow, deep breaths through your nose. Next, use your right thumb to gently close off your right nostril, then inhale slowly and deeply through your left nostril.

When you are ready to exhale, use your right ring finger to close off your left nostril while gently releasing the breath through your right nostril. Then switch the fingers you are using so that you are now closing off the left side with your right thumb and releasing the breath through your left nostril with your left ring finger. Repeat this pattern until you have finished practicing Nadi Shodhana Pranayama – 3-11 times, depending on how long you want to spend doing this exercise.

Remember to stay aware of both body and mind as you go through each step – notice any feelings of tension or anxiety beginning to fade away, and enjoy the rejuvenating sensations of calmness and clarity that invariably follow when you are done! Whether you are looking for stress relief or simply want to feel more mentally and physically balanced throughout the day, Nadi Shodhana Pranayama is a great way to achieve those goals without using complicated instructions or equipment.

2. Samaveta Pranayama

The Samaveta pranayama, or focused breathing, is a powerful breathing technique that has been used for centuries to help calm the mind, increase focus and concentration, and promote healing. To practice this technique properly, you must follow a step-by-step process that includes specific rhythmic patterns of inhalation and exhalation. Here are the basic steps for performing Samaveta pranayama:

1. Start by sitting still in a comfortable upright position with your eyes closed and your shoulders relaxed. Make sure your spine is straight, and your head is straight as well.
2. Take a few deep breaths, focusing on expanding your belly as you inhale and then gently compressing the air out of your lungs as you exhale. This will help to prepare your body for the next stage of breathwork.
3. Begin to focus on the natural flow of your breath; mentally count each inhalation and exhalation, holding it steady at five or six as you breathe slowly in through your nose and out through pursed lips. Stay in this rhythm as long as possible, working up to 10 minutes or more if desired.
4. When ready to finish the pranayama practice, slowly draw in a few last deep breaths through both nasal passages before exhaling fully out of both nostrils at once. Return gradually to normal breathing, taking note of any sensations you may feel in your body or mind during or after this exercise.

Regardless of how you feel afterward, remember that Samaveta pranayama carries many benefits when performed regularly over time!

3. Ujjayi Pranayama

Ujjayi pranayama, also known as the "victorious breath," is a great breathing technique for improving overall health and well-being. It involves long, slow breaths that are done in a specific way to maximize your body's oxygen intake. To perform ujjayi pranayama, you'll start either by sitting upright or lying down in a comfortable position. Next, focus your attention on gently relaxing any areas of tension in your body. You should then breathe slowly and deeply into your belly, using both the inhale and exhale to create a sense of balance between your body and mind. As you breathe in this manner, try to keep a gentle smile on your face and maintain total awareness of each breath. With practice, ujjayi pranayama can help you achieve peace, relaxation, and inner calm – making it an essential tool for healthy living.

4. Bhramari Pranayama

The Bhramari Pranayama technique is a powerful breathing exercise that can also be used to help calm the mind and relieve stress. To perform this practice, you simply need to take a comfortable seat, plug your ears with your thumbs, and begin to exhale slowly through your nose. As you do this, keep your mouth closed and gently vibrate your lips using the sounds "ohm" or "hum." Continue these steps for as long as you would like, taking mindful breaths throughout the process. Whether you are looking to reduce anxiety or simply find some much-needed clarity in your day-to-day life, this breathwork technique is an excellent tool that can help you achieve balance and well-being at any time.

5. Kapalabhati Pranayama

The Kapalabhati Pranayama technique is a popular breathing exercise that has been used for centuries to promote overall health. Taking just a few minutes out of your day to perform this type of breathwork can help improve your respiratory system, mental clarity, and digestion. To get started with this technique, follow these step-by-step instructions:

1. Begin in a comfortable seated position, with your spine straight but relaxed. Let your hands rest gently on your lap or your knees.
2. Inhale deeply through your nose, then exhale forcefully through your mouth while simultaneously pulling in your stomach and actively pressing out all of the air from your lungs. This movement should be smooth and controlled without any pausing between the inhale and the exhale. You should feel a light pressure pushing against your navel as you exhale.

3. After each forceful exhalation, pause briefly before taking another deep breath through the nose. At this point, you may also choose to pause at the end of each round of Kapalabhati breaths and take several normal breaths before starting again. Continue practicing until you feel calm and centered, focusing on relaxing your body with each breath cycle.

Whether you're looking to reduce stress or enhance your physical performance, the Kapalabhati Pranayama technique offers an excellent way to revitalize the mind and body through conscious breathing practices.

6. Anuloma Viloma

The Anuloma Viloma Pranayama, also known as alternate nostril breathing, is an excellent way to calm the mind, ease anxiety, and promote better sleep. This breathing exercise is simple to learn and can be done anywhere – making it a great tool to add to your self-care routine. This practice involves performing a specific sequence of steps to tap into the power of the breath and improve health and well-being. To get started with this technique, you'll need to find somewhere comfortable and quiet where you can focus on your breath. Then, follow these step-by-step instructions:

1. Begin by taking a few deep breaths, clearing your lungs, and preparing yourself for the practice ahead.
2. Inhale slowly through your nose, concentrating on drawing the breath deeply into your nostrils.
3. Hold your breath in for just a moment before exhaling slowly through your mouth, maintaining constant attention on the movement of air as it leaves your body. Try to visualize exhaling all negative emotions with each out-breath.
4. Repeat this process several times until you feel calm and centered, then continue practicing as desired to reap the many benefits of this powerful breathing technique.

7. Bhastrika Pranayama

Bhastrika is a powerful breathing technique used for thousands of years to boost energy levels, increase circulation, and improve overall physical health. This pranayama method is fairly simple to learn but does require some practice to perfect. Start by sitting in a comfortable position with your spine straight and your shoulders relaxed. You can sit cross-legged on the floor or on a chair with both feet planted firmly on the ground. Begin by taking a few deep breaths, filling your lungs, and then slowly releasing the air.

With each inhalation, draw the breath deep into your belly and feel it expanding your lower ribs as well. Pay special attention to any areas that feel tight or restricted, gently massaging them with each breath as you inhale and exhale. Next, take a moment to close your eyes and focus all of your attention on your breath. Begin by slowly and deeply inhaling through both nostrils for about four seconds, feeling the breath fill your abdomen from bottom to top as if it were an empty balloon rapidly filling with air. Then hold this breath in for another four seconds before slowly exhaling through both nostrils for about eight seconds, emptying all of the air from both lungs at once like squeezing out the water from a wet sponge.

And finally, hold the space for four seconds before repeating this round of breaths one more time – inhaling for four seconds and exhaling for eight seconds – at a slightly quicker pace than during round one. Continue doing these rounds of deep breathing 10 times, following this pattern:

> 4-4-8; 4-4-8; 4-4-8; 3-3-6; 3-3-6; 3-3-6; 2-2-4; 2-2-4; 2-2 -4;
>
> 1-second inhalation/1-second exhalation/4-second pause between breaths (rounds 1 through 5); 1-second inhalation/1-second exhalation/2-second pause between breaths (rounds 6 through 10).

Once you have reached ten total rounds of Bhastrika Pranayama, take five more slow deep breaths to physically relax your body before slowly coming out of this posture. And be sure to drink plenty of water after doing Bhastrika so as not to rid yourself of too much vital energy!

8. Sitali Pranayama

Sitali Pranayama is a technique that involves gently inhaling in a special breathing technique known as the rolled tongue breath. To perform the technique, you'll need to first form a small tube with your tongue by rolling it along the roof of your mouth. Once you have created the proper "tube," you can slowly inhale through your mouth, drawing in as much air as you can comfortably handle. As you inhale, focus on releasing any tension or stress that may be held in your body, allowing it to flow out toward the tips of your fingers and toes.

When you are finished with the inhalation, hold your breath for a few seconds before gradually exhaling through your nose. With each repeated cycle of this technique, try to focus on relaxing further and deeper within yourself. Over time, Sitali Pranayama can help to relieve stress and anxiety, leaving you feeling calm and refreshed. If you are interested in learning more about this ancient practice and how to get started right away, keep reading further for step-by-step instructions!

Pranayama is an incredibly powerful tool that can be used to improve your physical and mental health in manways. In addition to promoting relaxation and stress relief, pranayama can also help to improve your breathing, increase your energy levels, and boost your immune system. There are plenty of pranayama techniques that you can try depending on your needs and goals, so be sure to experiment until you find the one that works best for you. Remember to start slowly and gradually increase the length and depth of your breaths as you become more comfortable with the practice. Most importantly, have fun and enjoy the journey!

Chapter 7: Meditation Techniques to Try Now

One of the most common questions people have about meditation is, what is the point? Why sit still and focus on your breath when there are so many other things you could be doing?

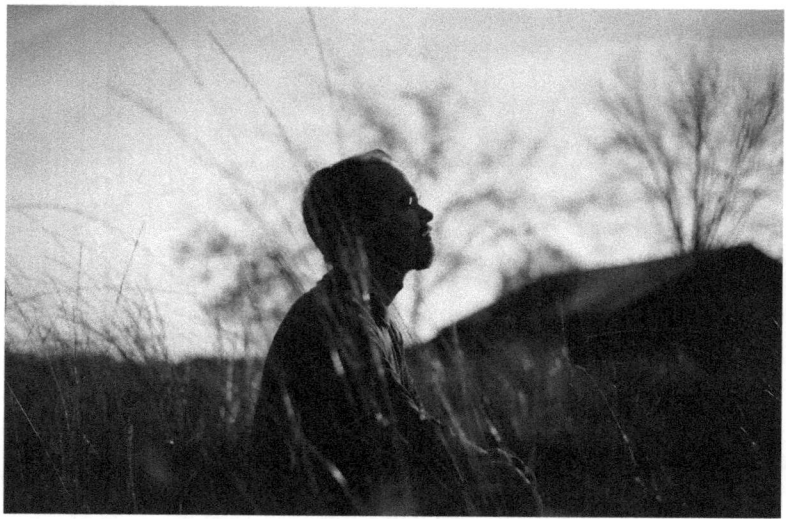

Meditation has been used for centuries as a way to achieve inner peace and gain a deeper understanding of the self.
https://www.pexels.com/photo/silhouette-of-man-sitting-on-grass-field-at-daytime-775417/

The answer to this question lies in the fact that meditation has been practiced for centuries by people from all walks of life. It is only in recent years that meditation has become popularized in the Western world. Meditation is an ancient practice that has its roots in many different cultures and philosophies. The goals vary depending on the tradition, but the common thread is that meditation is a way to focus and calm the mind.

There are many different ways to meditate, making it easy for you to find one you like and are comfortable doing. This chapter will explore the different types of meditation, as well as provide tips on how to make it a part of your daily life.

The Purpose of Meditation

Meditation has been used for centuries as a way to achieve inner peace and gain a deeper understanding of the self. In meditation, one gradually clears the mind of mental distractions and learns to focus instead on the present moment. Through this, we cultivate greater awareness, get insight into our thoughts and emotions, and find deeper meaning in our actions. And as we do it regularly, we can better understand who we truly are, connect more deeply with others, and experience life more fully and joyfully. These are the outcomes we want - to nourish our minds, bodies, and spirits so that we can live more meaningful, fulfilling lives.

Attaining turiya is the ultimate goal of meditation, though it takes time and effort to get there. Turiya, the fourth and highest state of consciousness, is a state of pure awareness beyond the three states of waking, dreaming, and deep sleep. When you meditate, your goal is to quiet the mind and reach a state of pure consciousness. In this state, you see things as they are, without the filters of your thoughts and emotions. You can connect with your true nature, which is pure love and peace.

Different Meditation Techniques

Many different meditation techniques can be used to achieve the state of turiya or ultimate oneness. One common approach is breath meditation, where you focus on your breath and simply observe any thoughts, emotions, or sensations that arise without trying to control or alter them in any way. Other popular techniques include awareness meditation, in which you pay close attention to every aspect of your experience as it unfolds moment by moment, and mantra meditation, where you silently repeat a word or phrase to yourself to gently redirect your train of thought when your mind starts to wander.

Whichever technique you choose, be consistent and practice regularly if you want to tap into the stillness and serenity that characterizes the state of turiya. Ultimately, what matters most is not so much the particular tools you use but rather your willingness to commit wholeheartedly to the meditative process itself. To discover for yourself what lies hidden beyond the veil of ordinary consciousness, all you need is the courage to take that first step.

20-Second Meditation

Meditation is a powerful tool that can help you stay focused, reduce stress, and gain greater insight into your innermost thoughts and feelings. One of the most effective is the 20-second meditation for Turiya. This technique involves building up to a state of deep, focused concentration over the course of 20 seconds, which then allows you to achieve a more relaxed and peaceful state during moments when you are otherwise stressed or distracted. The 20-second meditation can be done anywhere and at any time, making it a convenient and accessible way to bring more mindfulness into your day-to-day life.

To practice the 20-second meditation, find a comfortable place to sit or lie down. Close your eyes and begin focusing on your breath. Notice the sensation of the air moving in and out of your lungs. Then, start counting each inhale and exhale until you reach 20. Once you reach 20, allow your mind to become still and simply observe any thoughts or emotions that arise without judgment or attachment. With regular practice, this short 20-second meditation has the power to calm your mind and bring about lasting peace and clarity.

Aumkar Meditation

Aumkar meditation is a practice that can help you achieve the state of turiya or Cosmic Consciousness. Contemplating the sound of Aumkar can help to synchronize your mind and body with the rhythms of nature, allowing you to tap into deep levels of awareness and stillness. To get started with Aumkar meditation, begin by sitting in a comfortable position that allows your spine to be straight but not rigid. Close your eyes and take some deep, rhythmic breaths. Then, focus your attention on the sound of Aumkar as it vibrates through the air around you.

As you listen to this sound and allow it to fill your mind, try to let go of distracting thoughts and emotions that may arise. Stay present in the moment and remain focused on the experience of listening to Aumkar. Continue this practice for as long as it feels right for you, taking note of any insights or revelations that come up along the way. With regular practice, you'll be able to use Aumkar meditation as a tool for exploring deeper states of consciousness and ultimately achieving turiya – or ultimate peace and enlightenment.

Kundalini Meditation

Kundalini meditation is a powerful tool for achieving inner peace and spiritual awakening. The practice involves using focused breathing, chanting, and visualization practices to activate the body's energy centers or "chakras." In particular, the kundalini meditation technique involves directing the breath and awareness up through the body's central energy channel from the base of the spine to the highest chakra at the crown of the head.

To begin a meditation session, you'll need a comfortable sitting position with your spine straight but not rigid. Once you are settled in, you can start by taking several deep breaths through your nose and then slowly exhaling through your mouth. As you focus on each inhalation and exhalation, simply feel any sensations that arise in your body and mind. With each out-breath, repeat a phrase such as "let go" or "allow peace" until you feel ready to further engage with this meditation practice.

You can then move your attention to visualizing an imaginary line running up along your spine from your tailbone up to the crown of your head. As you picture this line, focus on activating each chakra along it by imagining them glowing bright red or gold as they come alive from inside. You can also chant short phrases like "Om Namah Shivay" or "Aum" for additional support as you move deeper into your meditative state. Continue focusing on these visualizations and sounds until you feel ready to finish up your kundalini meditation session. Then, take a few moments to gently bring yourself back into awareness of your surroundings before standing and moving slowly back into normal waking consciousness.

Transcendental Meditation

Transcendental Meditation (TM) is a unique form of meditation that has gained popularity in recent years. TM is simple and easy to learn, unlike other types of meditation, which often require intense concentration or deep introspection. To practice it, you simply follow a series of step-by-step instructions designed to guide your mind into a state of restful awareness called "Turiya."

The first step in learning TM involves identifying a mantra – a short word or phrase that helps to quiet the mind and focus your thoughts. You can either choose the mantra yourself or use one of the many mantras your teacher can give you. Once you have chosen your mantra, close your eyes and recite it quietly several times until you feel yourself letting go of any lingering distractions. Then, as you continue to repeat the mantra, you allow yourself to fall into deeper stages of restful awareness until, eventually, you reach Turiya.

That's all there is to it. With regular practice, this simple technique can help you achieve greater clarity and peace of mind, so you can experience life more fully and with greater joy. So if you're looking for an effortless yet powerful way to enhance your well-being, consider giving transcendental meditation a try today.

Zazen Meditation

Zazen, or Zen meditation, is a powerful practice that can be used to achieve inner peace and clarity. At its core, zazen involves simply sitting still and returning your awareness to the present moment. To get started with zazen meditation, first find a quiet place where you can sit undisturbed for a few minutes at least twice a day. Once you are in your meditative space, begin by taking a few deep breaths and focusing your mind on your breath as it flows in and out of your body. Once you feel more relaxed and centered, allow your awareness to expand beyond your physical senses. Continue to focus on the present moment as you allow thoughts, emotions, and sensations to arise and pass away on their own. With consistent practice, zazen meditation can help you reach a state of higher consciousness.

Mantra Meditation

Mantra meditation is a practice that can help you to achieve a higher state of consciousness. This technique involves focusing on your breath and repeating a mantra or phrase over and over again in your mind. While this might sound simple, there are several steps to follow to get the most out of this type of meditation.

The first step is to find the right mantra or phrase for you. Usually, this involves choosing a word or combination of words that have special significance or resonate with you on a deep level. You also need to find an appropriate tone - something soothing and relaxing, but not so bland that it becomes monotonous and distracting. Once you've found your mantra, start by repeating it softly in your mind as you breathe in and out, pausing regularly between each repetition if needed.

As you continue your meditation, try to focus all your attention on the sound and sensation of your breathing. Slowly, let yourself become more absorbed in the words of your mantra. As thoughts arise in your mind, simply acknowledge them and then return gently back to the rhythm of your breathing and the soothing sound of your mantra. With regular practice, you'll begin to experience deeper levels of awareness both during and after meditation sessions, ultimately reaching the state of turiya – a state beyond thinking, where only peace remains.

Mindfulness Meditation

Mindfulness meditation is a powerful tool that can be used to cultivate inner peace and promote overall well-being. This practice involves focusing your attention on the present moment without getting caught up in negative or distracting thoughts. As such, it can help to promote increased awareness, relaxation, and clarity of mind. In particular, mindfulness meditation is often used as part of turiya, which involves expanding consciousness to the point of enlightenment.

To practice mindfulness meditation for turiya, there are several key steps that you'll need to follow. The first step is to find a quiet and comfortable space where you can sit undisturbed for at least 10 minutes. You should then clear your mind and concentrate on your breathing, observing each breath as it flows naturally in and out of your body. Engaging in some gentle stretching exercises before beginning your meditation session may also be helpful if you feel tense or tight in any area of your body.

Finally, as you start to enter a deep state of relaxation during your session, do not let yourself fall asleep or get lost in a daydream – focus solely on being present during each moment. With regular practice, mindfulness meditation for turiya can help you access higher levels of consciousness and live a more peaceful and fulfilled life.

Body Scan Meditation

Body scan meditation is a popular mindfulness practice that benefits both the mental and physical health of those who practice it regularly. To do a body scan, one first needs to cast away all distractions and focus entirely on their body. This can be done either by lying down and relaxing the entire body from head to toe or sitting upright with one's attention focused on different areas of the body in turn. Throughout this process, it is crucial to keep your mind open, calm, and focused on the present moment.

As you begin your body scan meditation, start by focusing your attention on your feet. Slowly work your way up through each part of the body—calves, thighs, hips, stomach, breast muscles and organs, arms and hands—until you reach the head and face. Take note of any sensations that arise in each area while remaining detached from any emotions they may produce. Perhaps you'll feel some tension or discomfort in certain parts of your body; at these times, remember to simply accept what you are feeling without trying to fight it. Remaining mindful throughout every step will allow you to reap all the mental and physical benefits that this type of meditation has to offer. You'll be amazed at what a difference it can make!

Loving-Kindness Meditation

Loving-kindness meditation is one of the oldest and most popular forms of meditation out there. Also known as metta or Metta Bhavana, this practice involves tuning into loved ones and sending thoughts of kindness, care, and compassion their way. To begin a loving-kindness meditation for turiya, find a comfortable and quiet place where you can focus without distractions. Once you are settled in, take a few deep breaths to center yourself and clear your mind of any stresses or distractions.

Next, focus on someone that you feel love and gratitude toward - perhaps a friend or family member who has been especially kind or supportive. When you have found your object of attention, start by visualizing yourself sending this person love and good wishes. Feel the warmth of these feelings radiating out from your heart as you focus your attention on them. With each breath, repeat an intention for the other person's well-being: may they be happy and healthy, may they be at peace, and may they experience all the joys of this life and beyond. Continue focusing on these expressions of care until they feel like second nature.

Finally, bring in some extra energy and broaden your sense of compassion to include others in your life - maybe a mentor or beloved pet - who have also brought joy into your world. As you repeat the same intentions for their happiness and well-being, try to expand that feeling outwards so that it includes everyone around you - even strangers who may be going through difficult times. With each repetition, let go of any egoistic boundaries between yourself and others until all forms of suffering melt away like fog dispersing before the sun. And when all other thoughts pass by like clouds in the distance, stay in this state of loving-kindness - pure awareness free from constraint and change at all times with no beginning or end to existence itself.

Visualization Meditation

Visualization meditation is a powerful practice that can be used to achieve deep states of relaxation and consciousness. As with any form of meditation, start slowly and develop your skill over time. If you are new to visualization meditation, here is a step-by-step guide for getting started:

1. To begin, find a comfortable place to sit or lie down, somewhere where you will not be disturbed. Close your eyes and take a few deep breaths, focusing on each inhale and exhale.
2. Once you feel calm and centered, imagine that you are standing in an open field or meadow, surrounded by tall grass and trees. Notice the fresh green colors of the plants around you, as well as the gentle sounds of birds chirping or rustling in the wind.
3. Next, imagine that there is a bright ball of light directly in front of you. This is your inner light – the source of all compassion, wisdom, and insight within you. Slowly breathe in this beautiful light until your entire being feels surrounded by its warm radiance.
4. Now that you have established your inner light as a reference point for calmness and focus, spend some time visualizing this light streaming out from every pore of your body like a fountain of energy and awareness. Let go of any thoughts or worries as they arise in your mind, instead focusing all your attention on this brilliant white flow of light within you.

With patience and sustained practice, you'll soon be able to enter even deeper states of consciousness using visualization meditation techniques like these.

Making Meditation a Way of Life

The benefits of meditation are well-documented, ranging from improved mental and emotional health to enhanced spiritual growth. Yet despite its many benefits, many people fall into the trap of trying out meditation without having a clear plan for making it a regular habit. While adding meditation to your daily routine can be challenging at first, it's possible to successfully integrate it into your lifestyle by taking small steps that build upon each other over time. For example, you might start by setting aside a few minutes each morning or evening for sitting in stillness, gradually working up to longer periods as your body and mind become accustomed to the process.

In addition, you can make your practice more effective by setting goals, breaking larger goals down into smaller milestones, and engaging with others who share similar interests. With the right mindset and approach, meditation can quickly become a powerful tool for achieving greater happiness and well-being in your life.

Meditation is a simple but powerful tool that can be used to improve your mental and emotional health, as well as your spiritual well-being. While establishing a regular meditation practice may take some time, it is well worth the effort. By taking small steps and setting goals, you can make meditation a part of your daily routine and reap all the benefits that come with it.

Chapter 8: Useful Mantras and Mudras

Mudras and mantras are two important "accessories" to the practices of meditation and yoga. Mudras are hand gestures that help to focus and enhance awareness, while mantras are chanted words or phrases that also help to calm and focus the mind. Both mudras and mantras can be used to help attain the state of Turiya or the fourth state of consciousness. In this chapter, we will take a closer look at each of these accessories, including some of the most important mudras and mantras to know.

Mudras

Mudras involve using specific hand gestures to help facilitate movement and flow in the body. While many people associate mudras with physical postures, they can also be used as tools to enhance focus and awareness during meditation. To achieve turiya, the deepest state of meditation characterized by pure consciousness, mudras can be especially powerful.

One of the best-known mudras for turiya is called Shunya mudra, which is when you cup your hands at chest height and touch your thumbs together in front of your chest. This mudra helps to build energy at the third eye chakra between your eyebrows, boosting concentration and bringing clarity of thought. Other commonly used turiya mudras include maha bandha and Ardh Chandra Bhedana, each involving different hand poses that help activates different energy centers within the body to further deepen one's meditative state.

While these techniques are not a magic bullet for achieving turiya on demand, they can be useful tools to support deeper states of consciousness during meditation practice. So if you're looking to enhance your focus and awareness while going for turiya, consider incorporating some mudras into your practice!

Kali Mudra

This mudra is said to help access the fourth state of consciousness, known as turiya. Kali Mudra has many different meanings, depending on the context in which it is used. One of the most common interpretations of Kali Mudra is that it symbolizes strength and control over one's emotions.

- **Purpose**

The practice of the Kali Mudra is thought to help with a wide range of different health and wellness issues. Often used in yoga, there are multiple different theories about how and why this mudra works, but there is some evidence to suggest that it gives practitioners a sense of calm, improves circulation, and offers relief from joint pain. Whether you are looking for help dealing with chronic stress or simply want to find a way to improve your overall well-being, Kali mudra is an effective tool that can be adapted to meet your unique needs.

- **Symbolism**

Kali Mudra is a symbolic gesture; it serves as a representation of many different concepts and ideas. Kali represents both the destructive and creative powers of nature, while the open palm symbolizes the receptivity that comes with humility and trust. Moreover, crossed fingers are said to represent surrendering to one's true self or letting go of personal attachments. With these meanings in mind, it's easy to see why Kali Mudra is such a crucial gesture for practicing yogis. Whether you're seeking spiritual awakening or simply a moment of inner peace, this simple yet powerful mudra can help you on your journey to enlightenment.

- **Instructions**

To perform this mudra, you extend your hand outwards and bend your middle three fingers down towards your palm, keeping the thumb and ring finger straight. To use Kali Mudra in meditation, simply hold the gesture for a few minutes while quieting your mind. This can help to calm and center you, drawing focus inward to your inner self. Some people also use

Kali Mudra as a stress relief technique, taking deep breaths into their bent-down fingers to send calming energy throughout their bodies.

Whether you are looking for balance and grounding or simply seeking a moment of peace during a busy day, Kali Mudra can be an effective tool to help you achieve those goals. So, give Kali Mudra a try the next time you need a little help finding inner strength or regaining control over your emotions.

Jnana Mudra

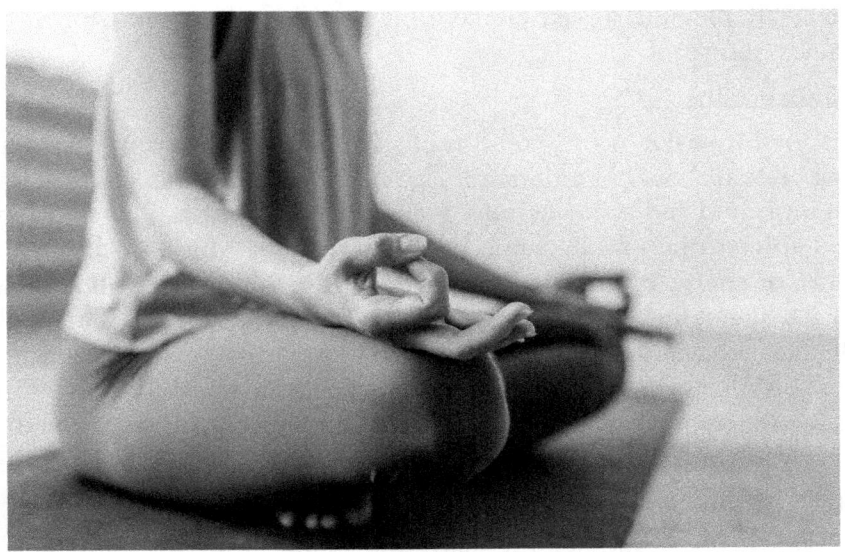

Jnana Mudra.
https://www.pexels.com/photo/a-woman-meditating-4534592/

Jnana is a Sanskrit word that means "wisdom" or "knowledge." This mudra is believed to have a variety of benefits, including improved focus and concentration, increased energy levels, and reduced stress.

- **Purpose**

The precise purpose of the gesture can vary depending on which school of yoga you are referring to. For instance, in some branches of yogic practice, the jnana mudra is thought to encourage the flow of energy along specific channels within the body, leading to greater vitality and well-being. In other traditions of yoga, the gesture is seen as a way to connect with higher states of consciousness or inner wisdom. Regardless of its precise meaning or function, one thing is clear: the jnana mudra has been gaining popularity in recent years as more and more people look for ways to enhance their meditation practice.

- **Symbolism**

Jnana Mudra is a symbolic hand gesture that has been used for centuries in various spiritual traditions, including yoga, Buddhism, and Hinduism. This iconic gesture is believed to be a symbol of knowledge and wisdom and can be used as a meditative practice or simply as an element of decoration. Jnana Mudra expresses a reverence for knowledge as a key component of spiritual growth. So whether you are using this mudra as a foundational part of your meditation practice or simply as an aesthetically pleasing design element, its meaning offers food for thought whenever you see it.

- **Instructions**

To perform the pose, you simply sit cross-legged with your hands resting on your knees in a mirror image of each other. This position forms the thumb and index finger into a circle while leaving the rest of your fingers spread open wide. Some people use Jnana Mudra to balance the chakras, or energy centers, in their bodies by focusing on specific points or areas when holding the pose. Other practitioners use it as part of their meditation routines to achieve greater levels of mental clarity and calmness. Whatever your reasons for practicing Jnana Mudra, this simple yet effective stance can help you to gain greater control over your mind and body as you relax into stillness.

Surya Mudra

Surya Mudra is another popular hand gesture. Surya means "sun" in Sanskrit, and this mudra is said to represent the energy and life-giving power of the sun. This mudra has a variety of benefits, including improved focus and concentration, increased energy levels, and reduced stress. Whether you are an experienced yogi or just beginning your journey into meditation, Surya Mudra is a simple but powerful tool for promoting well-being in body and mind.

- **Purpose**

Surya Mudra is a hand gesture that is commonly used in yoga and meditation practices. The purpose of this mudra is to help stimulate the energy centers of the body, - your chakras, by applying gentle pressure to specific points on the hands. By activating these energy centers, we can promote physical and mental health, reduce stress and anxiety, and enhance clarity of mind. With regular practice of this mudra, you can reap all the many benefits that it has to offer.

- **Symbolism**

Surya Mudra, also known as the "gesture of the sun," is an ancient finger pose with a rich heritage and powerful symbolism. This mudra is thought to be naturally energizing and warming, symbolizing both the sun's light and its life-giving power. According to traditional belief, practicing Surya Mudra can help revitalize your body, increase creativity, boost immunity, and awaken positive energy. Whether you practice this mudra as part of your daily yoga routine or simply as a way to center yourself during stressful times, it holds great potential for improving your mental, physical, and spiritual well-being. So why not go ahead and try out this simple yet meaningful meditative gesture for yourself? You might just be surprised by the benefits that it has in store for you!

- **Instructions**

The Surya Mudra is a simple hand gesture that can be used to improve circulation, reduce stress, and promote feelings of calm and well-being. This mudra involves placing the tips of your thumb and index finger together, giving the rest of your hand a loose and open appearance. To perform this mudra, simply sit comfortably with your hands in your lap or at your sides. Then, gently touch the tips of your thumb and index finger together, maintaining this position for five to ten minutes at a time. Not only is the Surya Mudra an easy way to increase overall health and well-being, but it can also be practiced anywhere - no special equipment or instruction is required.

Mantras

A mantra is a word or phrase that is repeated during meditation to enhance focus and awareness. During deep meditative states, such as Turiya, mantras can be extremely effective for clearing distractions and helping to direct the mind towards stillness. Some of the most common mantras are simple repetitions of a single word, such as "peace" or "calm," while others incorporate more complex linguistic patterns that engage both the intellect and the emotions. Whatever form it takes, a mantra is a focused tool that can help to clarify one's intention and deepen their meditative experience. So whether you are just starting or you are looking to take your practice to new depths, incorporating mantras into your daily routine can be an excellent way to enhance your ability to achieve Turiya.

Om Shanti Shanti Shanti

Om Shanti, Shanti, Shanti is a sacred mantra that is used to promote inner peace and connect with the divine. This mantra can be repeated in times of stress or struggle to help soothe the mind and calm the soul. Through its peaceful vibrations, this mantra helps to align us with the universe and connect us with our higher selves.

- **Pronunciation**

Pronounced "ohm Shahn-tee Shahn-tee," this mantra is made up of three Sanskrit words that can be translated to mean "peace," "calm," and "quiet."

- **Meaning**

This simple yet profound invocation is traditionally understood as a form of meditation on divine peace. This mantra can be used as a tool to help clear the mind, focus the senses, and cultivate a sense of inner calm. In addition, many yogis believe that repeating the Om Shanti Shanti Shanti mantra can help to bring forth one's inner light or energy, supporting one's journey toward higher levels of spiritual awareness.

- **Significance**

The mantra Om Shanti Shanti Shanti has healing properties, helping us restore balance and harmony within our bodies and minds. Whether you are looking for spiritual guidance or simply searching for a little peace in your life, chanting Om Shanti Shanti Shanti can be a powerful tool for finding tranquility and enlightenment. So if you're looking to reconnect with yourself and your true purpose, let this ancient mantra help guide you home. Om Shanti, Shanti, Shanti.

Aum Namah Shivaya

Aum Namah Shivaya is a sacred mantra that is used to honor the Hindu deity, Shiva. It is often repeated during meditation as a way to connect with Shiva's energy and receive his blessings. In addition, Aum Namah Shivaya is also used as a tool for self-purification, helping us to let go of negative thoughts and emotions that may be holding us back.

- **Pronunciation**

Pronounced "ohm Nah-mah shi-vie-yah," this mantra is made up of four Sanskrit words that can be translated to mean "I bow to Shiva."

- **Meaning**

Aum Namah Shivaya is a sacred chant that is typically used as a mantra in meditation and spiritual practice. The powerful Sanskrit words are thought to help bring the individual into a deeper state of awareness, helping connect with the divine forces at work in the universe. According to tradition, Aum Namah Shivaya reflects the beginning, middle, and end of all things. It is said to embody the primordial vibration of creation and represents both struggle and release. In many ways, these two opposing forces form the core of human existence: from birth to death, we fight and strive for progress even as we inevitably succumb to decline and decay. Despite this hard truth about life, Aum Namah Shivaya reminds us that peace and contentment can be found through liberation from our earthly suffering. Through repetition of these sacred words and deep focus during meditation, we can come one step closer to finding this peace within ourselves.

- **Significance**

Aum Namah Shivaya is an ancient Sanskrit mantra that is said to be positively charged with spiritual energy. This powerful mantra has been used for centuries for enlightenment, helping people connect with the divine and release their innermost desires. But perhaps its greatest significance lies in its capacity to create feelings of peace and calm within the heart and mind. One can access a deep sense of inner tranquility by chanting this sacred phrase, allowing one to confront life's challenges with optimism and clarity. So whether you are looking for a way to connect with your spirituality or simply seeking some much-needed peace and stillness in your life, Aum Namah Shivaya is sure to offer profound insight and healing.

So Hum

The So Hum mantra is a powerful tool for connecting with your inner wisdom and tapping into the profound wisdom of the universe. This mantra consists of three simple words–so, hum, and so–which represent the balance between the self and the greater whole. By repeating this mantra and bringing your full focus to the sound of each word, you can quiet your mind, open your heart, and connect deeply with yourself as well as with all beings everywhere. In this way, the So Hum mantra is a healing and transformative practice that has been used for generations to promote peace, insight, and understanding.

- **Pronunciation**

Pronounced "soh-hum," this mantra is made up of two Sanskrit words that can be translated to mean "I am that."

- **Meaning**

The So Hum mantra is foundational in the yogic tradition. Also known as the "I am" or "The Secret Sound," this phrase is used as an affirmation of one's divinity and connects the individual with their higher self. Its meaning can also be interpreted more broadly as a reminder to stay grounded, connected with the present moment, and focused on what's truly important in life. Whether you are practicing yoga or simply trying to quiet your mind and focus your attention, the So Hum mantra can be very powerful for calming your mind and finding clarity in even the most stressful circumstances. Ultimately, this ancient Sanskrit phrase embodies the essence of transformation and spiritual awakening, reminding us that we are always exactly where we need to be.

- **Significance**

The So Hum mantra is a key element of yoga and meditation practice. Also known as the primordial rhythm, this mantra helps to bring balance and alignment to mind, body, and spirit. Focusing our attention on the So Hum sound can help us still the mind, connect more deeply with our inner self, and move toward greater harmony and well-being. Furthermore, simply reciting the mantra can profoundly affect our energy levels and emotional state. Whether you are looking to quiet your mind during meditation or increase your sense of peace and contentment in your daily life, the So Hum mantra holds great power and significance.

Mudras and mantras are two powerful tools used for self-transformation and healing. Mudras are hand gestures that help direct energy flow within the body, while mantras are sacred words or phrases that have positive spiritual effects. Both mudras and mantras can be used to promote feelings of peace, calm, and well-being. When used together, they can be incredibly powerful when used for self-care and personal growth. If you want to improve your well-being, consider incorporating mudras and mantras into your daily routine.

Chapter 9: Yoga Sequences to Unlock Turiya

Creating a daily yoga practice can greatly improve your flexibility, strength, and overall sense of well-being. However, with so many different techniques to choose from, it can be difficult to know where to start. In this chapter, we will put together all of the various poses, breathing techniques, meditation methods, mantras, and mudras into complete sequences that can be done daily or several times a day. Doing these sequences regularly will help you to create a healthy mind-body-spirit balance in your life.

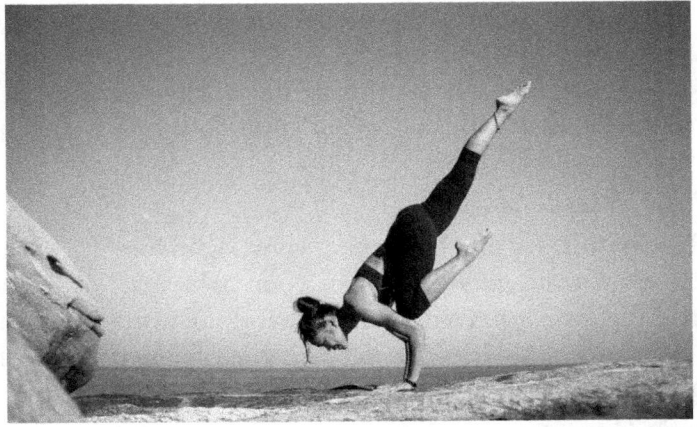

Creating a daily yoga practice can be a great way to improve your flexibility, strength, and overall sense of well-being.
https://www.pexels.com/photo/low-angle-view-of-woman-relaxing-on-beach-against-blue-sky-317157/

Monday Sequence

Starting your week off with yoga practice is a great way to set the tone for the rest of your week. This sequence will help you connect with your breath, center yourself, and release any tension you may be holding onto from the weekend.

Meditation Technique: Mindfulness Meditation

Begin by sitting in a comfortable position and focusing on your breath. Notice the sensation of the air moving in and out of your nose and lungs. Don't try to control your breath; just let it flow naturally. If your mind starts to wander, gently bring your attention back to your breath.

Breathing Technique: 4-7-8 Breathing

After you have finished your mindfulness meditation, do 4-7-8 breathing to help you relax. Breathe in for a count of four, hold your breath for a count of seven, and then exhale for a count of eight. Repeat this cycle several times.

Yoga Pose: Cat-Cow Pose

Start on your hands and knees in a "tabletop" position. As you inhale, drop your belly and look up towards the ceiling, letting your spine arch. As you exhale, round your spine up towards the ceiling and tuck your chin to your chest. Repeat this pose several times, moving slowly and smoothly with your breath.

Yoga Pose: Downward-Facing Dog

From your tabletop position, tuck your toes under and lift your hips up and back, coming into an "inverted V" shape. Straighten your legs as much as you can without compromising the natural curve of your spine. Let your head hang down and relax your shoulders. Stay in this pose for at least five breaths.

Yoga Pose: Warrior II

From Downward Facing Dog, step your right foot forward between your hands. Align your right knee over your right ankle and square your hips towards the front of your mat. Reach your arms out to the sides, parallel to the ground, and look over your right hand. Hold this pose for five breaths before switching to the other side.

Mantra: So Hum

After you have finished your Warrior II pose, come back to Downward Facing Dog and take a few deep breaths. Then, sit in a comfortable position and close your eyes. Repeat the mantra "so hum" to yourself silently. This mantra can be translated to mean "I am that" or "I am everything." Allow the mantra to sink in and just be with the feeling of it.

Mudra: Gyan Mudra

Finish your Monday sequence by sitting in a comfortable position and taking a few deep breaths. Place your hands in your lap with your palms facing up. Bring your index finger and thumb together to form a circle. This mudra is known as the "mudra of knowledge" and is said to promote concentration and clarity of thought.

Tuesday Sequence

On Tuesdays, we will focus on building strength and energy. This sequence includes some standing poses that will help to improve your balance and coordination.

Yoga Pose: Mountain Pose

Stand with your feet hip-width apart and your arms by your sides. Engage your core muscles and lift your shoulders up and back. Gaze forward and take a few deep breaths.

Yoga Pose: Half Camel Pose

From Mountain Pose, place your right hand on your lower back and reach your left arm up towards the ceiling. Gently arch your back and look up towards the ceiling. Hold this pose for five breaths before switching to the other side.

Yoga Pose: Chair Pose

From Mountain Pose, bend your knees and lower your hips down into a "chair" position. Keep your knees aligned over your ankles, and try to bring your thighs parallel to the ground. Reach your arms up towards the ceiling and hold this pose for five breaths.

Meditation: Body Scan

After you have finished your Chair Pose, find a comfortable seat. Close your eyes and take a few deep breaths. Starting at your feet, focus your attention on each part of your body and notice any sensations or emotions that you are experiencing. Don't try to judge or change anything; just observe and let go.

Mantra: Aum Namah Shivaya

When you have finished your body scan, sit for a few more minutes and repeat the mantra "Aum Namah Shivaya" to yourself. This mantra is a tribute to Lord Shiva, the Hindu god of destruction. It is said to promote peace and serenity.

Mudra: Ganesha Mudra

To end your Tuesday sequence, place one hand over the other, with the upper hand resting at the level of the heart. The thumb, index finger, and middle finger should all be touching, forming a triangle shape. The ring finger should be bent and pulled back, while the pinky finger should be extended and pointed outwards. By activating the Ganesha mudra, you can tap into your inherent inner wisdom to unlock your full potential on both physical and spiritual levels.

Wednesday Sequence

On Wednesdays, we will focus on flexibility and releasing tension. This sequence includes some gentle stretches that will help to release any tightness in your muscles.

Yoga Pose: Child's Pose

From a seated position, bring your knees up towards your chest and then slowly lower your hips back down to your heels. Rest your forehead on the ground and extend your arms out in front of you. Take a few deep breaths and hold this pose for as long as you like.

Yoga Pose: Cat/Cow Pose

From Child's Pose, move into an all-fours position with your wrists aligned under your shoulders and your knees aligned under your hips. As you inhale, arch your back and look up towards the ceiling. As you exhale, round your back and tuck your chin towards your chest. Continue this flow for a few breaths.

Yoga Pose: Pigeon Pose

From Cat/Cow Pose, bring your right knee forward and place it behind your right wrist. Slowly lower your left leg back and extend your right leg out behind you. You can place a blanket under your hips for support. Hold this pose for five breaths before switching to the other side.

Meditation: Loving-Kindness

After you have finished your Pigeon Pose, find a comfortable seat. Close your eyes and take a few deep breaths. Think of someone in your life who you love and send them thoughts of warmth, compassion, and love. Then, extend those same thoughts to yourself.

Mantra: Om Mani Padme Hum

When you have finished your meditation, sit for a few more minutes and repeat the mantra "Om Mani Padme Hum" to yourself. This mantra is said to be the key to enlightenment and is used as a prayer for compassion.

Mudra: Compassion Mudra

To end your Wednesday sequence, sit in a comfortable position and place your hands in your lap with your palms facing up. Bring your thumb and middle finger together while keeping your index and ring finger extended. This mudra is known as the "mudra of compassion" and is said to promote feelings of love and understanding.

Thursday Sequence

On Thursdays, we will focus on balance and centering ourselves. This sequence includes some standing poses that will help to improve your balance and coordination.

Yoga Pose: Tree Pose

From a standing position, move your weight onto your left foot and bring your right foot up to rest on your left thigh. Keep your hips squared and your arms at your sides. Take a deep breath and raise your arms overhead. Hold this pose for five breaths before switching to the other side.

Yoga Pose: Half Moon Pose

From Tree Pose, bring your right hand down to the ground and lift your left leg. Keep your gaze focused on a fixed point in front of you to help with balance. Hold this pose for five breaths before switching to the other side.

Yoga Pose: Warrior III

From Half Moon Pose, lower your left leg back down to the ground and bring your arms back by your sides. Shift your weight onto your right foot and lift your left leg behind you. Lean forward from the hips, keeping your back straight. Hold this pose for five breaths before switching to the other side.

Meditation: Centering

After you have finished Warrior III, find a comfortable seat. Close your eyes and take a few deep breaths. Focus your attention on your breath and let all other thoughts fall away. Stay here for as long as you like.

Mantra: Om Gam Ganapataye Namah

When you have finished your meditation, sit for a few more minutes and repeat the mantra "Om Gam Ganapataye Namah" to yourself. This mantra is a prayer to Lord Ganesha, the Hindu god of wisdom and new beginnings.

Mudra: Shankh Mudra

To end your Thursday sequence, sit comfortably and place your hands in your lap with your palms facing up. Bring your thumb and index finger together while extending your middle, ring, and pinky fingers. With your right hand, form a "C" shape and place the back of your hand on top of your left, forming a conch shell. This mudra promotes calmness and stability.

Friday Sequence

On Fridays, we will focus on twists and releasing any tension that has built up during the week. This sequence includes some standing and seated Twist poses that will help to stretch and relax your muscles.

Yoga Pose: Half Camel Pose

From a standing position, kneel on your mat with your knees hip-width apart. Place your hands on your lower back and lean back, letting your head fall back as well. Hold this pose for five breaths.

Yoga Pose: Seated Twist

From Half Camel Pose, sit up and bring your legs out in front of you. Cross your right leg over your left and place your right hand on the ground behind you. Place your left hand on your right knee and twist your torso to the right. Hold this pose for five breaths before switching to the other side.

Yoga Pose: Half Lord of the Fishes Pose

From Seated Twist, bring your legs back into Half Camel Pose. Reach your left arm up overhead and then twist your torso to the right, bringing your left arm down to the ground behind you. Look over your right shoulder. Hold this pose for five breaths before switching to the other side.

Yoga Pose: Revolved Triangle Pose

From Half Lord of the Fishes Pose, straighten your legs and move into Triangle Pose. Reach your right arm up overhead and your left hand down to the ground. Twist your torso to the right, looking over your right shoulder. Hold this pose for five breaths before switching to the other side.

Meditation: Release

After you have finished Revolved Triangle Pose, find a comfortable place to sit. Close your eyes and take a few deep breaths. Focus your attention on your breath and let all other thoughts fall away. Stay here for as long as you like.

Mantra: Om Namah Shivaya

When you have finished your meditation, sit for a few more minutes and repeat the mantra "Om Namah Shivaya" to yourself. This mantra is a prayer to Lord Shiva, the Hindu god of destruction.

Mudra: Aum Mudra

To end your Friday sequence, sit with your spine straight. Bring your hands to your knees with your palms up. Bend your index and middle fingers down to touch the base of your thumb. Extend your ring and pinky fingers.

Saturday Sequence

On Saturdays, we will focus on deep stretches and relaxation. This sequence includes some restorative yoga poses that will help to stretch and relax your muscles.

Yoga Pose: Child's Pose

From a kneeling position, lower your torso down to your mat and stretch your arms out in front of you. Rest your forehead on the mat and breathe deeply. Hold this pose for five breaths.

Yoga Pose: Pigeon Pose

From Child's Pose, bring your right leg forward and place it in front of you so that your knee is next to your right wrist and your ankle is next to your left hip. Your left leg should be extended straight back behind you.

Lower your torso down to the mat and rest your forehead on your mat. Hold this pose for five breaths before switching to the other side.

Yoga Pose: Sphinx Pose

From Pigeon Pose, lower your torso down to the mat and slide your left leg back so that both legs are extended straight behind you. Place your elbows under your shoulders and prop yourself up on your forearms. Hold this pose for five breaths.

Meditation: Visualize

After you have finished Sphinx Pose, lie down on your mat and close your eyes. Take a few deep breaths and begin to visualize a peaceful place. It can be somewhere you've been before or somewhere you've never been. Imagine all of the details of this place – the sights, the sounds, the smells. Stay here for as long as you like.

Mantra: Om Mani Padme Hum

When you have finished your visualization, sit up and repeat the mantra "Om Mani Padme Hum" to yourself. This mantra is a prayer to the Buddha of compassion, Chenrezig.

Mudra: Compassion Mudra

To end your Saturday sequence, sit in a comfortable position with your spine straight. Bring your hands to your heart center, with your right hand cupping your left. This mudra is known as the "mudra of compassion" and is said to promote feelings of love and kindness.

Sunday Sequence

On Sundays, we will take a break from our routine and focus on self-care. This may include taking a relaxing bath, reading your favorite book, or spending time with loved ones. Do whatever you need to do to recharge and rejuvenate yourself for the week ahead. Walking in nature, eating healthy foods, and getting enough sleep are also great ways to care for yourself.

Relaxing Bath: Add some soothing aromatherapy or add a few drops of lavender oil to your bathtub to help you relax.

Reading: Curl up with your favorite book and escape into another world for a while.

Time with Loved Ones: Spend time with family or friends, or reach out to someone you haven't talked to in a while.

Walking in Nature: Take a walk in the park or the woods and appreciate the beauty around you.

Eating Healthy Foods: Fill your body with nourishing foods that will make you feel good.

Getting Enough Sleep: Make sure you get enough sleep each night to help your body and mind rest and recharge.

These are just a few examples of the many different types of sequences you can do at home to improve your health and well-being. Remember to listen to your body and breathing, and let go of any expectations or goals you have for your practice. Just be present in the moment and enjoy the process. While it is important to challenge yourself, find what feels good for your body and do what you can to nurture your mind, body, and soul.

Chapter 10: Your Daily Steps Towards Turiya

To achieve Turiya, it is crucial to have a lifestyle that is dedicated to this goal. This means more than just meditating or doing yoga every day. It requires a change in mindset and a commitment to becoming aware of one's thoughts, emotions, and actions. While it may seem like a daunting task, making this change in perspective is essential to successfully reaching Turiya. There are many ways to begin this journey, but some key practices include self-reflection, mindfulness, and compassion. These three pillars will help to lay the foundation for a more conscious way of living that will eventually lead to Turiya.

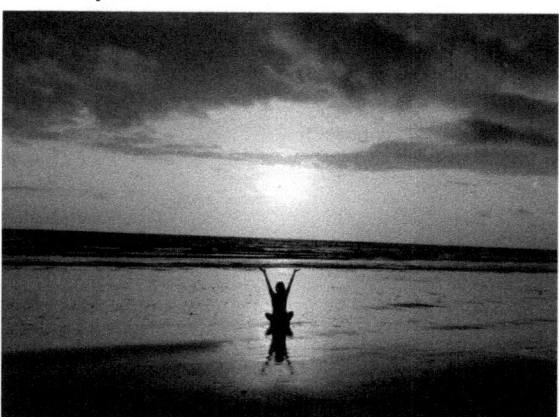

To achieve Turiya, it is crucial to have a lifestyle that is dedicated to this goal.
https://www.pexels.com/photo/silhouette-of-person-raising-its-hand-268134/

This chapter will give you a week-long schedule you can repeat to get closer to Turiya. Other than daily recommendations of meditation and yoga sequences, various other tips and tricks will be included, such as reminders to practice mindfulness, become aware of your consciousness, and get used to "becoming a witness" in your life. By following this schedule and implementing these tips, anyone can begin to live a more conscious and fulfilling life.

The Lifestyle of Turiya

Turiya is a lifestyle of peace and mindfulness. A key piece to this lifestyle is a devotion to creating inner awareness and equilibrium in all areas of life. Whether you are working, parenting, or simply taking a moment for yourself, Turiya encourages you to always be present and aware of the moment. This holistic approach means that you can enjoy everything from mindful eating and exercise routines to creative hobbies and social engagements while embracing an attitude of acceptance, appreciation, and relaxation. By viewing your life in this way, you are better able to live with joy, purpose, and fulfillment as you savor each experience as it comes. The more balanced you are on the inside, the better you'll feel on the outside.

Tips and Tricks for Achieving Turiya

To achieve turiya, or the state of pure, transcendent consciousness, you have to step out of your normal routine and make some key changes in your daily habits.

Diet

One of the most basic things to focus on is diet. Since turiya is a meditative state where you experience deep, natural peace and harmony, your diet should be high in nutrients that promote healthy mental functioning. This may mean cutting back on caffeine and foods that are high in sugar, both of which can have a counterproductive effect on the clarity of the mind.

Meditation and Yoga

No discussion of turiya would be complete without mentioning the importance of meditation and yoga. These two practices go hand-in-hand to achieve a deeper level of consciousness. Meditation helps to still the mind and bring about inner peace, while yoga helps to physically align the body and create balance in the mind-body connection. The goal is to reach a state of complete harmony between the two.

Mindfulness

Mindfulness is key to achieving turiya. It means being present in the moment and being aware of your thoughts, emotions, and actions. It may seem difficult at first, but with practice, it will become second nature. One way to be more mindful is to focus on your breath and use it as an anchor to bring you back to the present moment whenever your mind wanders.

Compassion

Having compassion is an essential ingredient in the recipe for turiya. This doesn't mean that you have to be a doormat or agree with everything everyone says, but it does mean that you should try to see things from other people's perspectives and always be respectful. By cultivating compassion, you'll be able to find common ground with others and build strong, lasting relationships.

Awareness

Paying attention is also necessary to reach a higher state of mindfulness. Be aware of your thoughts, emotions, and actions, as well as the thoughts, emotions, and actions of others. It may seem like a challenge at first, but with practice, it will become easier . . . and soon, second nature. The more aware you are, the better able you'll be to find balance in your life and live with purpose and fulfillment.

Becoming a Witness

One of the best things you can do to achieve turiya is to become a witness to your own life. This means watching your thoughts and emotions without judgment or attachment. It may sound easy, but in reality, it's quite difficult. The key is to practice detachment and focus on the present moment. By doing this, you'll see things more clearly and find balance in your life.

Acceptance

Last but not least, it's essential to accept yourself and others. This means accepting your thoughts, emotions, and actions as well as the thoughts, emotions, and actions of others. It may seem difficult at first, but with practice, it will become easier. The more you accept yourself and others, the more balanced you'll be in your life and the closer you'll be to achieving turiya.

Practice Self-Reflection

One of the best ways to achieve turiya is to practice self-reflection. This is all about taking some time each day to sit quietly and reflect on your life. What are your thoughts, emotions, and actions? How do they make you feel? What can you do differently to improve your life? By reflecting on these things, you'll be able to see things more clearly and make changes that will lead you to a more balanced and fulfilling life.

Visualization

Another great way to achieve turiya is to practice visualization. Take some time each day to sit quietly and imagine yourself in a state of complete harmony. Visualize that your mind and body are in perfect balance. See yourself surrounded by light and love. Fill yourself with positive energy and let it flow out into the world. By visualizing these things, you'll be able to bring them into your life and achieve a higher state of consciousness.

Prayer

Prayer is another powerful tool to help you achieve turiya. This means taking some time each day to connect with a higher power and ask for guidance. Pray for strength when you are feeling weak, courage when you are afraid, and wisdom when you are making choices. By praying for these things, you'll find them in your life and achieve a higher state of consciousness.

Connect with Nature

One of the best ways to achieve turiya is to connect with nature. Make time in your busy daily schedule to appreciate the beauty of the world around you. Notice the colors, smells, and sounds of nature. Feel the wind on your skin and the sun on your face. Take a deep breath and let the fresh air fill your lungs. By connecting with nature, you'll find balance in your life and achieve a higher state of consciousness.

Spend Time with Loved Ones

Spending time with loved ones is another great way to achieve turiya. This means taking some time each day to appreciate the people in your life. Talk to them, laugh with them, and just enjoy their company. Let them know how much you care about them. By spending time with loved ones, you'll find balance in your life and achieve a higher state of consciousness.

Be Grateful

Last but not least, be grateful for what you have. This doesn't mean that you should be content with your current situation, but it does mean that you should appreciate the good things in your life. By being grateful, you'll be able to attract more positive energy into your life and find balance and harmony.

Daily Recommendations

The previous chapter outlined a daily plan for achieving turiya. It's essential to have a daily routine that will help you stay on track. Here are some daily recommendations to help you get started:

1. Meditate for at least 10 minutes each day.
2. Make time for yourself to do things that you enjoy.
3. Eat healthy, whole foods.
4. Exercise regularly.
5. Get enough sleep each night.
6. Practice self-reflection.
7. Visualize yourself in a state of complete harmony.
8. Prayer for guidance.
9. Connect with nature.
10. Be grateful for what you have.

Achieving Turiya requires a lifestyle change dedicated to mindfulness and self-awareness. This can be a difficult process, but it is essential for reaching Turiya. The first step is to become aware of your thoughts and emotions. Be mindful of what you are thinking and feeling throughout the day. Pay attention to your reactions to situations and people. Notice when you are feeling stressed, anxious, or angry. These are all indications that your mind is not at peace.

The second step is to start making changes in your life to promote peace and relaxation. Begin by meditating for at least 10 minutes each day. Focus on your breath and let all other thoughts pass through your mind without clinging to them. Make time for yourself to do things you enjoy and make yourself feel good. This could include reading, spending time in nature, or practicing yoga.

The third step is to begin making changes in your diet and lifestyle. Eat healthy, whole foods that will nourish your body and mind. Avoid caffeine and alcohol, which can increase anxiety and stress levels. Exercise regularly to release tension and promote relaxation. Get enough sleep each night so that you feel rested and rejuvenated.

By following these steps, you'll be well on your way to achieving Turiya. Remember, it is a journey, not a destination. Take each day one step at a time, and be patient with yourself. Above all, enjoy the process.

Conclusion

In Hinduism, atman is the concept of the self, and turiya refers to the highest state of consciousness. In this state, the individual self is united with the absolute self. Turiya is a Sanskrit word meaning "the fourth" or "the highest." It is also known as pure consciousness, absolute consciousness, or the transcendental self. According to Hindu philosophy, there are four states of consciousness: waking, dreaming, deep sleep, and turiya. Turiya is the highest state of consciousness, in which the individual self is united with the absolute self. In this state, there are no distinctions between the subject and object, and all dualities are dissolved.

Many paths lead to turiya, such as yoga, meditation, and pranayama (breath control). Yoga is a system of physical and mental practices that originated in India. Meditation is a practice that allows the mind to become still and focused, and pranayama is a breathing technique that helps to control the breath. Mantras and mudras are also useful tools for inducing turiya. Mantras are sacred sounds believed to have spiritual power, and mudras are hand gestures often used in yoga and meditation. Yoga sequences can also be used to unlock turiya. These sequences are designed to open the energy channels in the body and prepare the mind for meditation.

There are many daily steps that you can take to move closer to turiya. Practicing yoga and meditation regularly is one of the best ways to achieve this state. Other steps include eating a healthy diet, spending time in nature, and connecting with like-minded people. By taking these steps and making a commitment to your spiritual practice, you can begin to experience the joy of pure consciousness.

Turiya is a state of pure bliss, peace, and unity. It is the highest state of consciousness that a human can experience. When you attain turiya, you'll feel a deep sense of connection to all that is. You'll also feel a sense of peace and well-being that is beyond words. This easy-to-follow guide helped you understand turiya and how you can experience it for yourself. It offered a step-by-step roadmap to help you understand this elusive but highly sought-after state and practice it in your life. Whether you're looking to improve your meditation skills or simply seeking more peace, clarity, and joy in your day-to-day life, this guide showed you how to find the inner stillness that lies at the heart of turiya. With just a little bit of time and effort, you can enjoy all the benefits of this timeless state for yourself.

Now that you have this knowledge, it is up to you to take the next step on your journey. Remember, the path to turiya is unique for everyone. Trust your intuition and follow your heart. And most importantly, enjoy the journey!

Here's another book by Mari Silva that you might like

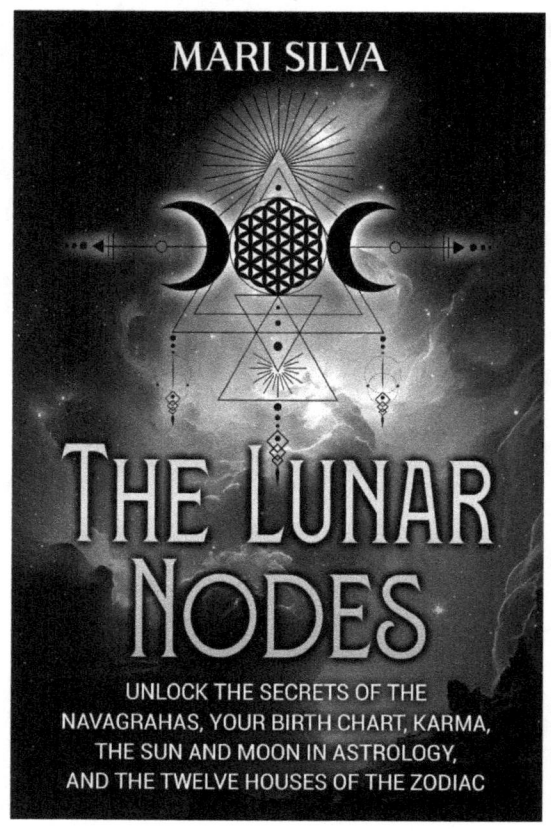

Your Free Gift
(only available for a limited time)

Thanks for getting this book! If you want to learn more about various spirituality topics, then join Mari Silva's community and get a free guided meditation MP3 for awakening your third eye. This guided meditation mp3 is designed to open and strengthen ones third eye so you can experience a higher state of consciousness. Simply visit the link below the image to get started.

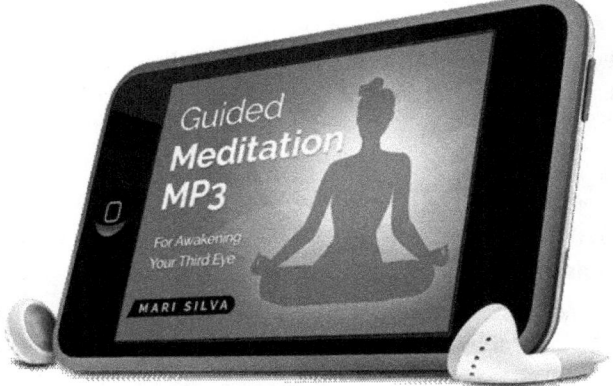

https://spiritualityspot.com/meditation

Or, Scan the QR code!

References

Fit, C. (2022, February 18). How to do Kriya Yoga: Meaning, type & health benefits of this ancient Yoga - blog.Cult.Fit. Cult.Fit; blog.cult.fit. https://blog.cult.fit/articles/kriya-yoga-learn-how-to-do-this-ancient-yoga-type-its-health-benefits

Kriya Yoga. (2013, February 9). Ananda. https://www.ananda.org/kriya-yoga/

Matson, M. (2020, September 20). What is Kriya Yoga? The Philosophy and Practice. Brett Larkin Yoga. https://www.brettlarkin.com/what-is-kriya-yoga/

Shroff, R. (2021, March 2). How to practice Kriya Yoga: Pranayama and meditation. MyYogaTeacher. https://www.myyogateacher.com/articles/kriya-yoga-pranayama-meditation

Steps to Kriya yoga. (2021, April 22). Ananda Sacramento - Yoga / Meditation / Community; Ananda Sacramento. https://anandasacramento.org/steps-to-kriya-yoga/

7 Chakras in human body, Significance & How to balance them. (2020, June 9). Art of Living (India). https://www.artofliving.org/in-en/meditation/meditation-benefits/seven-chakras-explained

Beaudoin, D. A. (2022, August 9). What is the subtle body? Yogajala. https://yogajala.com/what-is-the-subtle-body/

Bhakti, J. (2020, September 8). Prana, Nadis and chakras. Yoga Signs. https://yogasigns.com/prana-nadis-and-chakras/

Biernacki, L. (2019). Subtle body. In Transformational Embodiment in Asian Religions (pp. 108–127). Routledge.

Burton, N. (2021, December 5). How to unblock chakras: A complete guide to getting clear from root to crown. Goalcast. https://www.goalcast.com/how-to-unblock-chakras/

Everything you've ever wanted to know about the 7 chakras in the body. (2009, October 28). Mindbodygreen. https://www.mindbodygreen.com/articles/7-chakras-for-beginners

Jain, R. (2019, June 13). Complete guide to 7 chakras & their effects. Arhanta Yoga Ashrams. https://www.arhantayoga.org/blog/7-chakras-introduction-energy-centers-effect/

Lindberg, S. (2020, August 24). What are chakras? Meaning, location, and how to unblock them. Healthline. https://www.healthline.com/health/what-are-chakras

Love & Relationships. (n.d.). The complete beginner's guide to the seven chakras. Goodnet. https://www.goodnet.org/articles/what-are-seven-chakras-comprehensive-introduction

Matson, M. (2022, February 21). Awake in the subtle body: Yoga's 9th body. Brett Larkin Yoga. https://www.brettlarkin.com/the-subtle-body/

Muldoon, S. J., & Carrington, H. (2013). The projection of the astral body. Literary Licensing.

Prana. (n.d.). Yogapedia.com. https://www.yogapedia.com/definition/5154/prana

Prana and Chi Kung. (n.d.). Geneseo.edu. https://www.geneseo.edu/yoga/prana-and-chi-kung

Suri, K. (2020, January 22). Kriya Yoga: Spiritual progress through Kundalini awakening —. The Yogi Press. https://www.yogi.press/home/kriya-yoga

Trainer, A. J.-Q. (2022, March 18). The complete guide to the 7 chakras for beginners. Mindvalley Blog. https://blog.mindvalley.com/7-chakras/

Worldwide, A. S. (2018, July 10). Meditation & spiritual questions answered by expert yogis —. Ananda. https://www.ananda.org/ask/kriya-yoga-and-the-chakras/

Zoldan, R. J. (2020, June 22). Your 7 chakras, explained—plus how to tell if they're blocked. Well+Good. https://www.wellandgood.com/what-are-chakras/

Does Samadhi lead to Kundalini awakening? (n.d.). Quora. https://www.quora.com/Does-Samadhi-lead-to-Kundalini-awakening

Is kundalini awakening necessary for samadhi? (n.d.). Os.Me - A Spiritual Home https://os.me/community/spiritual-journey/is-kundalini-awakening-necessary-for-samadhi/

Seeker, S. (2020, October 9). What happens after Samadhi? Learnkriyayoga.com. https://www.learnkriyayoga.com/what-happens-after-samadhi/

Suri, K. (2020, January 22). Kriya Yoga: Spiritual progress through Kundalini awakening —. The Yogi Press. https://www.yogi.press/home/kriya-yoga

Worldwide, A. S. (2018, August 23). Meditation & spiritual questions answered by expert yogis —. Ananda. https://www.ananda.org/ask/samadhi-kundalini-awakening-and-more/

Ashish. (2019, April 4). What is Dhauti Kriya : 4 Types of Dhauti & Benefits. Fitsri. https://www.fitsri.com/yoga/what-is-dhauti

How To Make the Yamas and Niyamas Work for You in the modern world. (2018, January 15). Art Of Living (United States). https://www.artofliving.org/us-en/yoga/beginners/yamas-niyamas

Newlyn, E. (2015, June 7). The Yamas and Niyamas. Ekhart Yoga. https://www.ekhartyoga.com/articles/philosophy/the-yamas-and-niyamas

Tran, P. (2013, September 19). The yamas & niyamas in yoga. Everydayyoga.com. https://www.everydayyoga.com/blogs/guides/the-yamas-niyamas-in-yoga

Whittingham, R. (2019, November 24). What are the yamas and niyamas? Enjoy Yoga & Wellness. https://www.enjoycommunitywellness.com/enjoy-yoga-blog/2019/11/24/what-are-the-yamas-and-niyamas

Yaami, A. (2019, July 11). Vasti Kriya: 3 ways to cleanse intestine completely. Soul Prajna. https://soulprajna.com/vasti-kriya/

Yoga's ethical guide to living: The yamas and niyamas. (n.d.). Kripalu. https://kripalu.org/resources/yoga-s-ethical-guide-living-yamas-and-niyamas

Nunez, K. (2020, May 15). Pranayama benefits for physical and emotional health. Healthline. https://www.healthline.com/health/pranayama-benefits

Pranic energisation technique & jyothir trataka workshop - pradipika institute of yoga & therapy. (2020, July 24). Pradipika Institute of Yoga & Therapy. https://pradipikayoga.in/pranic-energisation-technique-jyothir-trataka-workshop/

SantataGamana. (2018, August 17). Kriya Pranayama. Real Yoga - Kundalini & Kriya Yoga Exposed. https://realyoga.info/2018/08/kriya-pranayama/

Shroff, R. (2021, March 2). How to practice Kriya Yoga: Pranayama and meditation. MyYogaTeacher. https://www.myyogateacher.com/articles/kriya-yoga-pranayama-meditation

YogaPoint. (n.d.). Pranayama. Yogapoint.com. http://www.yogapoint.com/info/pranayama.htm

Carver, L. (2020, October 6). 10 powerful meditation mudras and how to use them. Chopra. https://chopra.com/articles/10-powerful-mudras-and-how-to-use-them

Lowe, F. (2017, October 5). Motivate yourself with these simple mudras and mantras. Beyogi. https://beyogi.com/motivate-yourself-mudras-mantras/

Singh, A. (2021, February 4). Mudras & mantras to balance & awaken your chakras. Calm Sage - Your Guide to Mental and Emotional Wellbeing; Calm Sage. https://www.calmsage.com/mudras-mantras-to-balance-awaken-your-chakras/

Slocum, H. (2020, June 10). Meditating with mantras and mudras in therapeutic yoga —. PYI. https://www.premayogainstitute.com/pyi-blog/meditating-with-mantras-and-mudras-in-therapeutic-yoga

Van Fossen, Y. W. A. [YogawithAllieVanFossen]. (2021, August 4). 3 powerful mantras & mudras | how to stop stressing, overthinking & worrying. Youtube. https://www.youtube.com/watch?v=eVSQUjpGMr4

Acharya, T. (2018, May 14). Kriya Yoga Meditation. Nepal Yoga Home. https://nepalyogahome.com/kriya-yoga-meditation/

Fit, C. (2022, February 18). How to do Kriya Yoga: Meaning, type & health benefits of this ancient Yoga - blog.Cult.Fit. Cult.Fit; blog.cult.fit. https://blog.cult.fit/articles/kriya-yoga-learn-how-to-do-this-ancient-yoga-type-its-health-benefits

Gaiam. (n.d.). Meditation 101: Techniques, benefits, and a beginner's how-to. Gaiam. https://www.gaiam.com/blogs/discover/meditation-101-techniques-benefits-and-a-beginner-s-how-to

Hong-Sau technique of meditation. (2013, February 6). Ananda. https://www.ananda.org/meditation/meditation-support/articles/hong-sau-technique-of-meditation/

Learn Aum meditation technique —. (2013, February 6). Ananda. https://www.ananda.org/meditation/meditation-support/meditation-techniques/aum-technique/

United We Care. (2022, April 5). How to practice Om Mantra Meditation: A step-by-step guide. United We Care | A Super App for Mental Wellness. https://www.unitedwecare.com/how-to-practice-om-mantra-meditation-a-step-by-step-guide/

Asanas & kriyas. (2016, March 27). Shammisyogalaya.com. https://shammisyogalaya.com/yoga-asanas/

Moules, J. (2019, September 9). Practice these 7 Kundalini yoga poses and kriyas to focus your mind and balance your body. YouAlignedTM. https://www.yogiapproved.com/kundalini-poses-yoga/

Saanvi. (2018, March 13). Kriya Yoga Asanas and its Benefits. Styles At Life; Find the Information on Beauty, Fashion, Celebrities, Food, Health, Travel, Parenting, Astrology and more. Our Information is Highly confident and suggested Lifestyle Resources on the Internet. https://stylesatlife.com/articles/kriya-yoga/

United We Care. (2022, February 1). Kriya yoga : Asanas , meditation and effects. United We Care | A Super App for Mental Wellness. https://www.unitedwecare.com/kriya-yoga-asanas-meditation-and-effects/

Yoga poses: Sitting, standing, & recumbent Yoga Asanas for beginners. (2022, July 4). Art Of Living (India). https://www.artofliving.org/in-en/yoga/yoga-poses/sitting-standing-recumbent-yoga-poses

BrettLarkinYoga [BrettLarkinYoga]. (2017, September 20). Easy Kundalini Yoga practice for beginners (30-min) Kriya, poses, breath of fire, & meditation. Youtube. https://www.youtube.com/watch?v=-DO_GgchYPA

Hollister, S. (2018, March 23). Kundalini sequence to awaken the ten bodies. Yoga Journal. https://www.yogajournal.com/yoga-101/types-of-yoga/kundalini/kundalini-sequence-to-awaken-the-10-bodies/

Kaur, A. (2020, July 3). An introduction to Kundalini yoga sequences (Kriya). Serpentine. https://serpentine.yoga/an-introduction-to-kundalini-yoga-sequences/

Moules, J. (2019, September 9). Practice these 7 Kundalini yoga poses and kriyas to focus your mind and balance your body. YouAlignedTM. https://www.yogiapproved.com/kundalini-poses-yoga/

Beginner's guide: Paramhansa Yogananda's Hong-Sau Technique of Meditation. (2021, June 21). Kriya Yoga Home Study - Awaken Your Highest Potential. https://kriyahomestudy.org/technique-of-meditation/

Chakravarti, H. (2019, February 19). Breath and breath awareness. Kriya. https://harshavardhanweb.wordpress.com/2019/02/19/breath-and-breath-awareness/

Fellowship, S. E. L. (2018, May 10). Kriyayoga meditation. Self Enquiry Life Fellowship. https://hansavedas.org/kriyayoga/

Hellicar, L. (2022, September 16). What Is yogic breathing? Benefits, types, and how to try. Medicalnewstoday.com. https://www.medicalnewstoday.com/articles/what-is-yogic-breathing

Marjariasana: Benefits, steps. (2019, June 20). Wakefit | Blog. https://www.wakefit.co/blog/marjariasana-yoga-better-sleep/

Message, M. (n.d.). Pranayama: Samaveta pranayama - lesson 2.6. ASHLEY CRUZ YOGA. http://www.ashleycruzyoga.com/blog/pranayama-samaveta-pranayama-lesson-26

Mill Churning Pose. (2012, July 17). Art Of Living (Global). https://www.artofliving.org/yoga/yoga-poses/mill-churning-pose

Nagendra, P. by. (2016, June 9). crow walking Kawa Chalasana 8 – Learn Self Healing Techniques Online. Selfhealingonline.com. http://selfhealingonline.com/offer-item/crow-walking-kawa-chalasana-8/

Nanda, A. (2020, October 22). Ardha baddha konasana- half-butterfly pose- practice, benefits and contraindications. Moksha Mantra; Aashish Nanda. https://www.mokshamantra.com/ardha-baddha-konasana/

Pathare, S. (2016, June 22). 5 pranayamas that you should make a part of your daily fitness schedule. HealthifyMe. https://www.healthifyme.com/blog/5-pranayamas-make-part-daily-fitness-schedule/

Roderick, B. (2022, September 18). Simha Kriya the lions yawn. Dahn Yoga. https://www.dahnyoga.net/techniques/simha-kriya-the-lions-yawn.html

Russel, K. (2010, December 17). Kriya yoga – pranayama techniques. Yoga in Daily Life. https://pureyoga.wordpress.com/2010/12/17/kriya-yoga-pranayama-techniques/

Saithalyasana (Animal relaxation pose): Benefits, Steps and Precautions. (n.d.). MyUpchar. https://www.myupchar.com/en/yoga/legs/saithalyasana-animal-relaxation-pose-benefits-steps

Sarpasana (Snake Pose)– benefits, adjustment & cautions. (2018, March 6). Yoga India Foundation. https://yogaindiafoundation.com/sarpasana-snake-pose/

Shashankasana : Pose of moon or hare Pose. (2014, May 30). Yoga Ananda | Yoga for Happiness; Yoga Ananda. https://www.yogaananda.net/shashankasana-pose-of-moon-or-hare-pose/

Shroff, R. (2021, March 2). How to practice Kriya Yoga: Pranayama and meditation. MyYogaTeacher. https://www.myyogateacher.com/articles/kriya-yoga-pranayama-meditation

Simkhada, S. (2020, February 14). Methods of pranayama and swaasa Kriya. Himalayan Yoga Academy. https://himalayanyoganepal.com/methods-of-pranayama-and-swaasa-kriya/

Sukhasana - the easy sitting pose. (2014, May 28). Yogic Way of Life. https://www.yogicwayoflife.com/sukhasana-the-easy-sitting-pose/

United We Care. (2022, February 1). Kriya yoga : Asanas , meditation and effects. United We Care | A Super App for Mental Wellness. https://www.unitedwecare.com/kriya-yoga-asanas-meditation-and-effects/

Vyas, M. K. (2018, August 3). Gatyatmak Meru Vakrasana (dynamic spinal twist) yoga for stiff back and spine flexibility. MKV Yoga; Mahendra Kumar Vyas. https://mkvyoga.com/gatyatmak-meru-vakrasana-dynamic-spinal-twist/

Yoga Postures - Hip Rotation. (n.d.). Healthandyoga.com. https://www.healthandyoga.com/html/yoga/asanas/hip_rotation.aspx

Borohhov, D. (2011, May 28). Turiya meaning. Ananda. https://www.ananda.org/yogapedia/turiya/

Chitrapuri. (2012, February 25). Shiva and Shakti. Chakras.net. https://www.chakras.net/yoga-principles/shiva-and-shakti

Darecki, Y. (n.d.). Turiya. Com.au. http://yogananda.com.au/g/g_turiya.html

Durand, K. W. (2008). Turiya: A Collection of Wordizms. AuthorHouse.

Hughes, A. (2020, January 29). Shiva and Shakti: The divine energies within us all. Yogapedia.com; Shiva and Shakti: The Divine Energies Within Us All. https://www.yogapedia.com/shiva-and-shakti/2/6052

Purohit, T. (2022, February 3). Shiva and Shakti - the divine union of consciousness and energy. TemplePurohit - Your Spiritual Destination | Bhakti, Shraddha Aur Ashirwad. https://www.templepurohit.com/shiva-shakti-divine-union-consciousness-energy/

The. (2017, August 7). Turiya: The fourth dimension of being. The Tribune India. https://www.tribuneindia.com/news/archive/lifestyle/turiya-the-fourth-dimension-of-being-448113

The Editors of Encyclopedia Britannica. (2021). samadhi. In Encyclopedia Britannica.

Turiya of the fourth state. (n.d.). Sivanandaonline.org. https://www.sivanandaonline.org/?cmd=displaysection&section_id=752

VivekaVani [VivekaVani]. (2021, March 25). Turiya in Vedanta - Pravrajika Divyanandaprana. Youtube. https://www.youtube.com/watch?v=2LIxwolSDJw

www.ingramcontent.com/pod-product-compliance
Lightning Source LLC
Chambersburg PA
CBHW051854160426
43209CB00006B/1292